# TEST ANXIETY NO MORE

## A SIX-STEP GUIDE FOR COLLEGE AND GRADUATE SCHOOL EXAM SUCCESS

**Dr. Bianca Busch**

# Table of Contents

# Introduction

It's the winter quarter of freshman year at the University of Chicago during midterm season. The paper for General Chemistry—Variant B (a course tailored to doctors and scientists) lands on my desk: three pages with three questions and no multiple-choice safety net.

As I look over the questions, the blank spaces waiting for my answers stare back at me, expecting me to fill their void with principles and equations. The first two questions look familiar to me, and I'm confident I'll manage them. Question three, on the other hand... Well, let's tackle questions one and two first.

My confidence builds while I work on the first two questions, and I feel good about my answers. And then, I get to question three. As I read through it, I think I remember the information they're asking for. *Do I remember? Did we even cover this problem set in class?* As doubt creeps in, my memory starts to betray me. And worst of all, some of the students have already turned in their exams, looking confident about how they did.

I begin writing down my answer, but I pause and erase it. Write again, erase again. The paper seems to get thinner every time I put my pencil on the page. *Oh no! Maybe, I can write something that will at least give me partial credit?*

I check the clock. Only 20 minutes left. I felt the panic start to creep in as soon as I began working on this question, but now, it wraps its claws around my chest and my mind, making it harder and harder to think.

I glance at my peers, and their composure makes me more anxious. Only 10 minutes left. I quickly write down what I can, hoping to receive at least partial credit for attempting to answer the question.

With the examination over, I turn in my paper and flee, hoping to avoid any discussion about the test.

My anxiety is overwhelming at this point. All I can think is that surely, I failed. And if I had stayed to listen to everyone else talking about their answers and the exam, it would have been too painful.

Our grades are posted days later. I bundle up, hoping to ward off the biting Chicago wind, and trudge from my dorm at Burton-Judson to the basement of Kent. In 2006, our grades were posted on paper, so I had no choice but to make the trek across the midway and withstand the cold lake winds.

After arriving in the basement, I scan the list for my name. I can't remember the exact percentage, but my score hovered between 50 and 60%—physical evidence of my in-exam failure. Feeling helpless and unable to do anything about it, I turn around and make my way back to my dorm, tears stinging my eyes as I brave the cold and try very hard not to think about my results and the disappointment that's welling up in my chest.

I had graduated fifth in a class of almost 300 students at a public high school in Albuquerque, New Mexico. When I arrived at the University of Chicago, it was a dream come true. From the moment I stepped foot on campus, I was brimming with confidence in my academic abilities, convinced that I'd be able to ace my coursework just like I did in high school. And with scholarships and accolades paving my way, further fueling my belief in my abilities, all I could think was, *I can't possibly fail.* Until now.

Many people had told me that the University of Chicago would be a great place to deepen my learning, but nothing could have truly prepared me for what I was getting myself into. Sure, I knew the school's reputation. But I didn't yet understand what their uncompromising commitment to academic rigor meant for me.

On top of that, I quickly began to realize that many of my peers had been prepared in elite environments that made the transition from high school to university much smoother. Students formed informal study groups, and their familiarity with the rigor of this kind of academic environment far exceeded my own. Doubts and panic about my academic abilities and skills began to creep in. This was the moment my confidence first started to falter and anxiety began to take root.

While I'm now a board-certified psychiatrist who has trained at some of the nation's finest institutions, I still remember this defining moment in my academic career. My goal is to use my experiences and what I learned in overcoming my struggles with anxiety—along with my expertise as a psychiatrist—to guide you on your journey to overcoming your self-doubt and anxiety so that you too can reach your true potential.

You may have already had a similar experience to mine, but you don't have anything to be ashamed of. Test anxiety can be debilitating and can take down even the most well-prepared and talented student. That doesn't mean you can't take back control and overcome your foe, though.

You may be used to being told to simply "calm down" or "take some deep breaths" when you tell someone you're feeling anxious about an upcoming test. They may even tell you that you're smart and have prepared well, so you don't have anything to worry about. As well-intentioned as their words may be, they don't make your anxiety magically go away. If anything, you may feel even more frustrated, powerless, and overwhelmed. After all, they're unintentionally dismissing your very real anxiety and the impact it has on your mind and body.

So, how do you combat the fear and anxiety that occurs during tests and exams even after preparing for long periods? Are there specific strategies you can use to prepare and manage your anxiety? And can you adapt these tools to meet your specific testing needs?

The simple answer is yes! The longer answer is that this book is going to provide you with a variety of tools. You will learn how to overcome the feelings of overwhelm and anxiety that accompany various types of tests and exams.

This also includes learning how to take proper care of your mental and physical health since preparing for tests can make it easy to neglect your other needs. As this impacts your well-being, it's important that you learn how to achieve a balance between taking care of yourself and preparing for tests. By taking good care of your mental and physical health, you can make the preparation and learning process less overwhelming. You'll also feel more mentally and physically comfortable when taking the test.

When you walk away from this book, you will have the six steps you need to overcome your test anxiety and achieve your dreams. These steps include tools and strategies that can be easily adjusted to meet your specific needs and lifestyle. These techniques will give you the confidence to approach any type of test, exam, or presentation with confidence in your knowledge and abilities—which is helpful for any surprise quizzes, questions, or conversations you may encounter during your schooling and professional career.

Throughout this book, you'll also learn that you aren't alone in your struggles. Many people experience test anxiety at different ages, from young children to adults. Seeking help from a professional, like a counselor or therapist, can be really helpful. Professionals can give you insight into your anxiety, provide you with additional tools, help you apply them, and offer you support during difficult moments.

Thankfully, the practices that you'll discover in these pages will also benefit you throughout your life since they're incredibly adaptable. This means that you will be able to endure and overcome any obstacle or situation that triggers your anxiety using these steps, tools, and strategies. After all, anxiety may be a normal part of life, but that doesn't mean it should prevent you from achieving your dreams.

Before we dive into the strategies and tools that you will need for this journey, let's take a look at the importance of asking for help, as well as how you can do this in a way that meets your specific needs. Turn the page and start your journey to overcoming your test anxiety.

Chapter 1:

# The Value of Asking for Help

As a college student trying to navigate young adulthood and prepare for the rest of my life, I wasn't aware of what was actually going on both around and inside me. While I persevered and improved my test-taking abilities thanks to my experience as a post-baccalaureate student at a Harvard Extension School, my academic struggles returned almost as soon as I started medical school.

My first course was Anatomy, and I was quickly thrust into a completely new learning environment. But I still started out really excited about the course and what we would learn. After being assigned to my group for the class, I spent the majority of my time, both in and outside the lab, studying.

This meant a lot of late nights with cadavers. As creepy as it was, I wasn't alone, and I was determined to put in the work to succeed. I even attended practice quizzes hosted by upperclassmen. And then, the day of the exam arrived.

I started my day feeling confident and prepared. For the Anatomy test, we had to move from body to body and identify different muscles, tendons, and organs. We were also asked to occasionally go beyond identification and recite important supplemental information about their structures. That's when that old, familiar anxious feeling began to creep in.

My thoughts began to waver, and soon, I started to doubt myself. *I think this is the right name. Probably. Oh no! There's the timer. I have to move on.*

The spiral continued as I took the exam, and I kept doubting my knowledge and skills. My fear over whether I answered the previous question correctly harmed my ability to move on to the next section too. But I just couldn't stop thinking about it. Then, a thought that I think many of us are familiar with began to arise: *Oh man, I don't think I'm going to do very well on this exam, even after all the hours I spent studying and preparing. I can't believe this happened again!*

The smell of formaldehyde had been clinging to my skin for months. During preparation, I kept telling myself it would be worth it. Taking the exam, however, I was no longer so sure. This only added to my frustration. What if I had to take the exam again?

At this point, I had to consciously remind myself that I was still taking the exam and needed to finish it before planning for the future, but my anxiety was overwhelming. Self-doubt filled every stroke of my pencil, and my thoughts were clouded, making it hard to think.

I barely passed the Anatomy block with a C. I should have been happy. After all, I passed! But after the long hours and all the hard work I put in, I felt helpless. Something wasn't right, and while I recognized this, I didn't know how to put it into words.

After the results were released, many of us ventured on a camping trip to the Arches in Utah to celebrate the end of Anatomy. However, I still knew I needed to ask for help so that this didn't happen again. So, before we left for our trip, I reached out to the school's academic support specialist. Little did I know that this was just the beginning of my journey to figuring out how I learn best and how this knowledge would help me overcome my academic anxiety.

Nowadays, you may be taking your tests, exams, and assessments on a computer, but you're probably still quite familiar with this scenario. Though the testing environment has changed over time, that doesn't mean your test anxiety has lessened. If anything, you're now hovering your cursor between options A and B, hesitant to make a choice because you can't really be sure that you're right. Maybe, the answer is "all of the above." And the timer that counts down your online exam is probably just as frustrating and scary as a physical clock in a classroom—if not more so, since it's harder to avert your eyes from something on your screen.

If you're anything like me, you've already followed all of the recommended steps for preparing for your exam too. You read the textbook and worked through the material, took several practice tests, completed the problem sets, reviewed and reworked them, and maybe even asked your professor for tips on how best to prepare. If you're preparing for the professional entrance exams, then you've taken the Kaplan or Princeton Review Course too.

So, you know the material; there's no doubt about that. However, you may still be struggling to perform the way you should after all the hard work you've put in. I understand this, and it's a pain and frustration that's hard to put into words. The impact it has should still be taken seriously, though.

We're often expected to ask for help without being taught *how* to ask for help. And asking for help is a vital skill that everyone should have, especially if you struggle with anxiety. One of the many reasons asking for help is valuable is because it can help you obtain the tools and information you need to overcome obstacles and cope with the challenges that arise from your test anxiety in a healthy way. So, how do you develop this skill?

## Should You Ask for Help?

Test anxiety doesn't sound very serious until you're the one experiencing it. Those who have never felt this type of anxiety to the extent we have may even believe that you're simply nervous. But test anxiety is more than nerves, and it has its own pros and cons too.

One advantage of this type of anxiety is that it can keep you motivated and help you prepare properly for upcoming assessments and presentations. On the other hand, when test anxiety begins to interfere with your ability to think clearly during the situations that trigger it—preventing you from carrying out even the simplest task with your usual ease—it can begin to seriously affect your mental and physical well-being, leading to additional problems in your academic, personal, and professional life.

Experiencing debilitating test anxiety means that you are no longer able to go about your daily life as you normally would. So, not only does your anxiety become disruptive, it also makes life more challenging than it should be. Seeking help from a professional is particularly important in cases like this since test anxiety will affect your ability to think and concentrate, making learning, preparation, test-taking, and a whole host of tasks more difficult. You may also experience physical manifestations like high blood pressure and digestive problems. That's because the human body was never meant to exist in a state of constant stress and anxiety.

Purposefully seeking help from a mental health professional like a psychiatrist or counselor—depending on your needs and the resources you have access to—allows you to work with someone who is skilled and knowledgeable about identifying test anxiety and its impact on your life. They can help you manage and work through your anxiety to decrease its impact on your well-being and life.

As you can see, test anxiety's impact isn't limited to your grades. It doesn't have an age limit either. Around one-third of Americans have been found to struggle with anxiety at some point in their life (Berg, 2023). You aren't alone, and you have nothing to be ashamed of.

Seeking help is a sign of strength. After all, you would never have gotten to this point had you not been strong enough to endure anxiety's impact on you and your life. You don't have to continue suffering.

You deserve to have the information, tools, and skills to manage your anxiety so that you can enjoy your academic career and work toward your dreams. Seeking help from a professional is simply a healthy strategy that helps you achieve this. But what happens when you leave your anxiety untreated?

## *Impact of Untreated Anxiety*

Since anxiety can act as a motivator for preparing for tests, the question of whether you should treat your anxiety may have passed through your mind. Your schedule for school is probably already full, in addition to all your regular responsibilities, so you might be wondering if you should really be trying to take time to work on your anxiety too.

Yes! You opened this book because you know that you shouldn't be struggling this much while taking tests after having put in so much effort to prepare. Whether you seek professional help or work on your anxiety by yourself, intentionally managing your anxiety is crucial for your overall well-being, academic success, personal relationships, and ability to enjoy your life.

When your anxiety is left untreated, even for short periods, you may start to feel like you're being held back by some invisible force. The things you enjoy and the goals you're working toward may seem even more out of reach than they originally did, and you might start avoiding any situation that triggers your anxiety.

This could lead to additional problems like procrastinating exam preparation, avoiding study groups, isolating yourself from your peers and mentors, and missing opportunities. You may also begin experiencing additional mental health issues like depression.

Some individuals resort to unhealthy coping mechanisms to manage their anxiety. The use of alcohol, tobacco, cannabis, opiates, and even prescription medication are a few common examples. Since they don't have the knowledge or tools to manage their anxiety safely, the use of these substances contributes to additional problems like overdose and addiction, despite it not being the user's intention.

So, you have to ask yourself if staying in your comfort zone and avoiding your anxiety triggers is worth the life you are missing out on. I know this process isn't as easy as it sounds, but when left untreated, test anxiety can have a big impact on you and your life. The first step in the process of asking for help is understanding why you might be struggling to seek out guidance from experienced and qualified individuals.

## *Why Do You Struggle to Ask for Help?*

We all have our own reasons for struggling to ask for help, but there are a few common factors that contribute to this obstacle. Anxiety itself, for instance, can be a stumbling block when aiming to ask for help. So, how does this process work when you need help managing your anxiety, but you're too anxious to seek help?

We'll take a more in-depth look into anxiety, how it works, and how it impacts us in the next chapter. For now, you have to keep in mind that anxiety is a complex mechanism that is meant to keep us safe when we perceive threats in our environment. Taking tests and asking for help may not kill us, but the stress that they evoke can cause our minds and bodies to see them as threats.

Understanding that you feel anxious because your mind perceives the activity as potentially dangerous—even though you know you aren't in any physical danger—is the first step. It helps you remove some of the uncertainty surrounding this situation so that you can prepare yourself to complete the activity despite your anxiety.

This empowers you to have a better idea of the type of coping mechanisms that might help you manage your anxiety around a given scenario. For example, having a basic set of steps to follow when asking for help can make this specific situation less scary. Preparing yourself can make this process less overwhelming. It doesn't matter if you are seeking help from a mental health professional or asking your friend to help you out with a few daily tasks until you can attend your appointment, the preparation process can be easily adjusted.

It's also important to understand that challenges surrounding asking for help can arise because society has made us believe, from an early age, that we should all be able to handle everything on our own. However, this simply is *not* true.

Human beings are meant to support and rely on each other. Forming communities is normal because it naturally provides the support and stability we seek without making us feel like a burden or putting us in anyone's debt.

Seeking help provides you with access to communities of individuals facing similar struggles. If you join these communities, in addition to your session with your counselor or therapist, you'll learn that you're not alone in your struggles, and this can make managing your anxiety less overwhelming.

Asking for help doesn't mean you're a burden either. Oftentimes, mental health professionals enter this field because they want to help others, so they won't see you as a burden. Likewise, your friends and family won't see your request for help as bothersome. Friendship is built on mutual support; by asking for help, you are proving to your loved ones that they are trusted and valued members of your circle. Show yourself compassion too. Imagine that you are your best friend asking for help. Would you tell your friend they're a burden, or would you want to help them because you care about them?

Treating yourself as if you were your friend is a strategy that helps us remember that we're human and we don't have to be perfect. This makes it easier to show ourselves compassion and patience when we are struggling or make mistakes—which can be especially important if you're facing new or severe academic challenges.

However, not knowing how to ask for help or what may happen after seeking help can be scary. It's okay to be afraid when asking for help, but don't let that stop you from seeking the help you need. Sometimes, you have to do the hard thing that you know will help you despite being afraid. Knowing what benefits you may experience by seeking help can offer motivation to push through that fear.

## The Benefits of Asking for Help

Understanding what happens when you don't learn to manage your anxiety using healthy coping mechanisms and seeking help is important, but it may make you worry even more. Anxiety is a tricky adversary, so knowing as much as possible about it will equip you to successfully manage it in a way that meets your needs. In this section, we'll take a look at the advantages of seeking help.

### *Healthier Coping Strategies*

When you don't know that you're struggling with anxiety or don't know how to manage it properly, you may resort to unhealthy or dangerous coping mechanisms. This isn't anything to be ashamed of. You're doing the best you can with the tools you have. However, seeking help gives you the opportunity to use specific tools and strategies that add to your life and benefit your mental and physical health.

### *Decreased Risk of Additional Problems*

By seeking out help from a mental health professional, you can prevent or manage additional health problems. If you have a current underlying physical health condition that may be worsened by your anxiety, your mental health provider can work with you alongside your regular healthcare provider to minimize this risk. This is crucial if you have to take medications for your anxiety in addition to medications for your health condition. Managing your test anxiety can also provide you with overall health benefits like improved digestive health and better sleep quality.

### *An Opportunity to Connect With Others*

Managing anxiety isn't always a visible battle. Many of the people in your life may not even realize that you're struggling. This can make managing your anxiety a lonely experience. Seeking help from a professional allows you to connect with someone who understands what you're going through, helping you feel less alone and providing you with access to a supportive and uplifting community of individuals facing similar issues.

### *Better Relationships*

Maintaining and building relationships with other people can be hard when you're also trying to cope with your anxiety. This impacts your ability to network and connect with mentors and individuals in the professional field you're trying to enter too. Seeking professional help gives you the tools to work through these barriers so that when you interact with others, you can engage in productive conversations.

Asking for help may not always be given the same level of importance as other healthy coping mechanisms, but it truly is a valuable tool—one that can improve your overall well-being and quality of life.

## Step 1: Getting Help

There are many different ways you can go about asking for help. In this section, you'll find basic guidelines that will allow you to seek help despite your anxiety:

- You may feel uncomfortable about the thought of asking for help, but do it anyway. The long-term benefits of this activity will be worth the discomfort you feel right now.
- Self-criticism, negative thoughts, and assumptions can add more obstacles to this process without us even realizing it. Take a deep breath, and recognize that while you may have these assumptions about asking for help, that doesn't mean they're true. Recognizing and labeling them can help you take away some of their power and make it less overwhelming or scary to seek guidance.
- Determine who you want to ask for help. Friends and family are people you may trust, and talking with them can ease your anxiety, but you may also need to seek professional help. Mental health professionals have the expertise and knowledge to guide you through managing your test anxiety in a way that meets your unique needs.
- Recognizing that you're struggling and need help is an important step, even if you aren't sure what you need help with. Mental health professionals will have the knowledge and

experience to help you determine exactly what you're struggling with and what tools may benefit you.

- Consider all your options. There are many in-person and online mental health services available, and your university or college may have mental health services you can use.

### *Additional Tips*

- Remind yourself that you don't have to have everything figured out. You can ask for help without knowing exactly what type of guidance or assistance you need.
- If you find it difficult to verbalize your need for help, write it down, perhaps in the form of an email or text. This technique helps individuals who struggle to verbalize their experiences and emotions to communicate effectively with their mental health professionals.
- Reach out to a hotline or crisis line. They're available 24/7 and can provide you with support during moments when you're struggling but can't contact anyone else.

Asking for help isn't a complicated process, but it does have its challenges. However, it's crucial that you don't let this prevent you from seeking guidance from qualified professionals. Getting this far on your journey to overcoming your test anxiety is a sign of your strength.

## Key Takeaways

You probably relate to the experiences and struggles I've shared, and you've likely sought out this book because you haven't yet achieved your academic goals or are struggling to reach them despite all the effort you've already put in. You also know that your anxiety may be the main obstacle getting in your way.

Test anxiety has a bigger impact on your well-being and academics than you may realize, but it can be conquered through the use of evidence-based techniques like the ones that will be discussed in later chapters.

In addition to building your own healthy coping patterns, it's also important that you ask for help. Personally, I could not have overcome my academic struggles without seeking help and guidance. So, while you can embark on this journey on your own, asking for help could be a crucial first step to overcoming your anxiety and beating your testing blocks. Additional takeaways from this chapter include

- recognizing that you have experienced academic success in your life, and it's possible that you will again.
- understanding that even when you put in the work to prepare for your exams—by completing the homework and working through the preparation courses—you may still be struggling.
- realizing that it is possible to conquer your academic anxiety.
- understanding that evidence-based help is available and that your journey to using these strategies successfully begins in this book.

Your goal may be to use the steps in this book solely as a method to help you prepare for your next exam. But consistently putting in the work and using the tools to help you manage your anxiety will benefit you throughout your life. After all, increasing your comfort level while taking exams could lead to professional advancement and, later on, success and fulfillment in your life—outcomes that also result from the type of work you want to do.

Throughout this book, we're going to look at some of your deeper thoughts which likely affect other areas of your life too. You'll explore different aspects of your identity so that you can learn how to calm and manage anxious feelings as they arise, no matter where you are in life.

Anxiety is a natural part of our lives, but it doesn't have to be overwhelming. There will be moments when your anxiety rises to distressing levels in areas of your life besides academics. With the tools and steps from this book, you'll be prepared to handle these challenges. This means that you'll have the skills to identify when you're feeling anxious and do something about it, allowing you to live your life calmly and confidently. Now that we know how to ask for help, we can move on to more deeply understanding anxiety and its impact on our lives.

## Chapter 2:

# Understanding Your Test Anxiety

Feeling anxious is an experience we have all shared at one point in our lives. This is probably why you can easily relate to someone who says they're feeling anxious regardless of the situation or event that is causing them to feel that way. You have to keep in mind, however, that like any human circumstance, the way you experience anxiety may differ slightly compared to others. Regardless of how your test anxiety manifests, your experience is valid. Recognizing that your test anxiety can show up in a way that's unique to you and your situation provides you with valuable information for managing it effectively.

Nevertheless, anxiety, like other mental health conditions, can generally be recognized by a specific set of signs and symptoms. While they may manifest in different ways, at varying intensities, the impact they have on your well-being is generally similar to the impact they have on others.

This level of similarity from person to person is also true of the triggers of anxiety. For example, you could be in university taking exams on anatomy while another person may be in high school taking their math test, and you could both struggle with test anxiety. That's because one of the biggest triggers of test anxiety is the physical act of having to prepare for and take a test, regardless of the testing conditions, environment, type of exam, subject, or your age.

So, while the exact details of the triggers and causes of test anxiety—as well as other anxiety conditions—may differ between individuals, its impact on your mental and emotional well-being can be very similar. These commonalities create the foundation needed to truly understand your test anxiety, its origins, what could trigger it, and how it might be affecting you and your academic career.

This information empowers you to adjust the tools and strategies for managing your test anxiety so that they better suit your needs, experiences, and lifestyle. While you and anyone else who reads this book will be making use of the same exercises, your individual experiences, answers, and the way you implement them will differ. But this doesn't make them any less effective.

Don't compare yourself or your experiences to other people who struggle with test anxiety, as your situation will be unique. The tools that work for you may also need to be adjusted differently to work for someone else. Connecting with others who experience test anxiety can help you to recognize that each person takes their own path to healing, ensure that you feel less alone on your journey, and provide you with support and connection. Remember that even if you haven't been in the same situation as your peers, your experience and the impact test anxiety has is still valid.

You aren't alone on your journey, and you deserve to use the tools and strategies discussed in this book to take back control of your life. One of the best ways to get started, besides seeking professional support, is to understand what it is you're up against.

## What Is Anxiety?

You already know that you're struggling with test anxiety, so why are we discussing anxiety on its own? Well, this mental health condition impacts many people all over the world, and test anxiety is only one of many types of anxiety a person could struggle with. It's also important to understand that, unlike certain types of anxiety, test anxiety isn't officially recognized as its own condition by the Diagnostic and Statistical Manual of Mental Health Disorders, Fifth Edition (DSM-5).

This is important to understand since the DSM is the medical reference book used by professionals and experts to understand, study, classify, and diagnose brain-related and mental health conditions like ADHD, depressive disorders, and anxiety disorders.

While test anxiety may not be categorized as its own condition, it is considered a manifestation of other anxiety conditions. This is also why it's crucial to seek out professional guidance. An expert, like a psychiatrist or psychologist, can ensure that you don't have an underlying anxiety condition that also needs to be cared for.

By taking a look at what anxiety is in general, we're able to better understand what test anxiety is, how it could be affecting different areas of your life, as well as its impact on your overall well-being.

In general, anxiety is known as a natural and adaptive response that occurs when you are stressed out or perceive a threat. That's because the brain is wired to ensure your continued survival, allowing for the development of certain life-saving responses that we don't always have control over, like the fight-or-flight response.

This response is a type of anxiety reaction that occurs when you perceive or notice a danger to your continued safety. Adrenaline—one of several chemical messengers and hormones in the body—is released at the start of this response to prepare your body to react quickly, resulting in specific physical, behavioral, and cognitive changes that aim to keep you safe. Life-threatening and stressful situations, like a car accident or physical attack, are potential triggers of the fight-or-flight response. But presentations, social situations, and taking exams can likewise trigger an anxiety reaction.

Since an anxiety reaction like the fight-or-flight response is meant to keep us safe, we can recognize that not all anxiety is bad. In fact, anxiety is a very normal human experience. That's why almost everyone has been able to say that they've felt anxious before.

Problems start to arise, however, when your anxiety begins to become excessive and persistent. Your anxiety may begin to interfere with your daily functioning, making tasks that you never struggled with before challenging. When this happens, it is considered an anxiety disorder. The following list contains three examples of anxiety disorders that people experience:

- **Social anxiety disorder:** caused by a fear of rejection, humiliation, and judgment by strangers and people you know when you are in public or during a social situation.

- **Generalized anxiety disorder:** characterized by long-lasting symptoms of anxiety whose trigger may not be limited to a single event, situation, or cause.

- **Specific phobia:** when your uncontrolled feelings of anxiety are triggered by a specific situation or object, like spiders, and you can acknowledge that your reaction, fear, and avoidance of it is extreme or illogical, but you still experience the related feelings regardless.

Remember that test anxiety hasn't been included in this list because it's not officially recognized as a distinct condition by the DSM-5. That doesn't mean it should be taken less seriously since this form of anxiety can still have a serious impact on your well-being, life, relationships, and performance on tests. Let's take a closer look at what test anxiety is.

### *Test Anxiety*

We know that it's normal to experience fear and anxiety before, during, and after an exam, presentation, or other testing situation. The degree to which you experience these emotions is often manageable and will allow your mind to stay alert, helping you perform well on the test without your cognitive abilities becoming impaired.

However, these feelings of anxiety can become so extreme that they start to interfere with and impair your ability to perform during the testing situation, preventing you from performing to the best of your abilities. This combination of emotional reactions and physical symptoms that negatively affect your test-taking abilities is what is known as "test anxiety."

While this type of anxiety may not be officially recognized in the DSM-5, it should still be taken seriously because it's more than a bit of worry before and during the test or exam; it's impairing your ability to perform your best on a test regardless of how much or how little preparation you've put in, and it can manifest in disruptive ways before, during, and after the test.

This could explain why test anxiety can also be viewed as a type of performance anxiety. However, there are several potential triggers of test anxiety.

### *Fear of Failure*

A common contributor to test anxiety is a fear that you will fail regardless of the amount of work you've put in. This fear can occur for many reasons, including connecting your sense of self-worth to the outcome of the tests you take. This only adds extra pressure and stress, in addition to the regular nerves you already experience before an upcoming test.

### *Poor Testing History*

While you may often do well on tests, any past failure or difficulties during testing may contribute to your current anxiety. In this case, test anxiety arises because you're afraid of experiencing the same situation or results, as well as the negative emotions experienced during that situation.

### *Biological Feedback Loop*

The physical symptoms of anxiety, which we will discuss in the next section, can become so severe and uncomfortable that they make it even more challenging for you to focus. They can trigger extreme physical discomfort that causes your already struggling mind to become even more distracted. These symptoms may also impact your cognitive abilities, making it even more challenging for you to focus and further exacerbating your fears.

From your own experiences with anxiety, you've likely already realized that it can affect you in many ways. You may even notice that certain symptoms arise during your classes or study group sessions, while also occurring alongside more intense symptoms during the actual testing situation.

In the next section, we'll look at the signs and symptoms of test anxiety so that you can continue to develop your understanding of the impact this condition can have on your overall well-being and test-taking abilities.

## Signs and Symptoms of Test Anxiety

At moderate levels, anxiety can help you become more alert. This is a useful trait when you need to focus and concentrate during tests; it may even help you perform better on exams and during presentations. But as we now know, higher levels of anxiety can start to interfere with your overall performance.

This occurs because when your levels of anxiety start to increase, emotional, physical, and cognitive symptoms will begin to manifest. As their severity increases, your mental and cognitive functioning will start to become more and more impaired. You can get a better idea of how these symptoms might manifest and impact you using the three categories that follow.

### *Cognitive Symptoms*

Several mental behaviors could indicate you're struggling with test anxiety. Negative self-talk, self-doubt, memory problems, intrusive thoughts, racing thoughts, blanking out, and feeling overwhelmed and helpless are a few common cognitive symptoms related to test anxiety.

I always struggled with a flood of negative thoughts like, *I don't know enough*, *I'm not prepared*, and *I'm not going to do well on this exam*. These thoughts would manifest despite all the hard work and time I had put in to prepare for every test. Sometimes, I also struggled with my mind going completely blank, making an already stressful testing experience even more terrifying.

### *Physical Symptoms*

You're likely already familiar with a few of these symptoms but shaking, dry mouth, sweating (particularly in palms and armpits), headache, nausea, shortness of breath, rapid heartbeat, fainting, vomiting, muscle tension, and diarrhea (among other gastrointestinal issues) are physical signs of test anxiety.

### *Emotional Symptoms*

When you know you have an upcoming test, you may experience several emotional signs that your test anxiety has been triggered. These symptoms often include several negative emotions, like feelings of hopelessness, depression, anger, frustration, low self-esteem, and irritability.

You may even notice that these unpleasant experiences result in additional behaviors, like skipping class or avoiding study groups and preparation sessions. While you know you need to prepare or attend these groups, you may avoid them to prevent yourself from having to experience the unpleasant flood of negative thoughts, emotions, and other physical symptoms that often accompany test anxiety.

I understand just how challenging and painful test anxiety can be. Before and during tests, my heart used to beat really fast, and my palms were so sweaty I struggled to hold my pencil during the exam. Short bursts of nausea and feeling like I was on the edge of vomiting were also common. When I reflected on these signs while working on managing my test anxiety, I also realized that I would roll my neck from side to side and shrug my shoulders in hopes of relieving the muscular tension that would set in when my anxiety was triggered.

The symptoms of test anxiety can be experienced to various degrees. This means that these symptoms can become intense enough to trigger additional problems too. Panic attacks are one such example. So, how do you tell the difference between severe anxiety and a panic attack?

## Are You Having a Panic Attack?

The first time I had a panic attack, I thought that something was very wrong with my body. It happened suddenly. I couldn't breathe, and my chest was becoming concerningly tight. All I could think was, *Do I need to go to the emergency room?*

At the time, I was living in Allston, Massachusetts, just outside of Boston, in a big Victorian house. I had six—yes, *six*—roommates, and thankfully, one of them was nearby when the panic attack hit. They helped me breathe through it and sat with me until the symptoms began to subside.

Yet, I still felt like something was very wrong. I followed up with my doctor and demanded an electrocardiogram (EKG). This test helps healthcare providers record the heart's electrical signals, information that's valuable when trying to determine whether someone is having a heart attack or suffers from an irregular heartbeat. And the symptoms I had experienced during the panic attack were ones that I had, up until that moment, associated only with heart attacks. So, I must have had a heart attack, right?

Fortunately, my heart was found to be in top shape. After speaking with my doctor, I learned that I had had a panic attack. This was shocking because how could something as simple as panicking about a test manifest in such intense physical symptoms? It quickly made me realize just how big of an impact test anxiety can have on the mind and the body.

Having dealt with panic attacks before, I now understand just how scary they are in the moment. They make you feel like you've lost all control, and you may even believe that you're dying despite not being caused any physical harm. While I obviously didn't enjoy having panic attacks, they did provide me with the opportunity to understand what my own patients go through. That's also a comfort to the patients I've worked with since I know exactly how they feel and what they've experienced.

But why are we talking about panic attacks? The symptoms of test anxiety can become intense enough to culminate in a panic attack. Panic attacks are extremely scary to experience, especially if you are on your own. Intense and overwhelming feelings of fear and discomfort come on very suddenly and are often accompanied by four or more physical symptoms.

Panic attacks are often unexpected, making them even scarier, and they can happen to anyone. Take note that the repeated occurrence of panic attacks can result in a panic disorder and, due to their intensity, often require professional treatment.

These attacks can also be tricky because they can occur without having a specific trigger. All we can be sure of is that this panic is connected to anxiety in general. So, if you learn to manage your test anxiety effectively, you'll lower your risk or number of panic attacks.

While my own experiences with panic attacks provide insight into how it feels, let's still take a deeper look at the distinguishing symptoms of panic.

### *Physical Symptoms*

- rapid heartbeat
- shaking or trembling
- tightness or pain in your chest
- numbness and tingling in your toes and hands
- suddenly feeling very hot or very cold regardless of the actual temperature
- sweating even when it's cold

- feeling like you're choking or can't breathe
- feeling as though you're moments away from vomiting
- dizziness, unsteadiness, or fainting

### *Psychological Symptoms*

- overwhelming feelings of fear
- a sense of impending doom or belief that something catastrophic will happen soon
- feeling disconnected from your reality, like your surroundings or the situation isn't real
- worrying that you're going crazy or losing control of yourself
- experiencing a flood of worries and fears that make it difficult to focus on one thought
- a fear that you're dying

These symptoms may appear suddenly and without warning. Their intensity generally peaks within 10 minutes of starting, but they can last up to half an hour. Once the attack has ended, you'll likely feel drained and exhausted.

Knowing the signs of a panic attack equips you with a better understanding of what's going on in your body. This makes it easier to prevent and manage them in the future. For example, if you experience mainly physical symptoms, then your coping skills should focus on promoting bodily relaxation.

Interestingly, panic attacks and test anxiety share symptoms. As such, they are often confused despite not being the same thing. Let's look at the difference between these two conditions.

### *Panic Attack Versus Anxiety Attack*

Sometimes, people use the terms "anxiety attack" and "panic attack" interchangeably, but they aren't the same thing. Anxiety attacks aren't recognized as a formal condition or experience and don't have specific diagnostic criteria, unlike panic attacks. Instead, severe anxiety is recognized as contributing to anxiety-related disorders that manifest as symptoms that can interfere with your ability to carry out tasks or perform during social and testing situations.

Panic attacks, on the other hand, cause physical and emotional symptoms that appear very suddenly and intensely compared to the symptoms of anxiety. So, how do you figure out if you're experiencing severe anxiety or having a panic attack?

#### *Tips for Telling the Difference*

- Panic attacks don't always have a specific trigger or stressors, while test anxiety will have identifiable triggers.
- Anxiety can be experienced at varying intensities, while panic attacks don't normally have different intensities. They are a sudden, intense, and overwhelming experience overall.
- Panic attacks can occur as a single episode. Anxiety, however, can last for long periods, and its symptoms can vary in intensity during this time.

Test anxiety and panic attacks can both occur as a result of your fears and concerns regarding tests. Fortunately, there are many evidence-based strategies and tools you can use to tackle your test anxiety and prevent it from turning into a panic attack. The six steps outlined in this book will provide a pathway to reducing your anxiety and mitigating your risk of panic attacks.

I know that the six steps work because I've used them to help me manage my own test anxiety. After performing poorly in Anatomy, I started exploring my learning needs. One of the most crucial parts of this journey was working with a therapist to understand my test anxiety, but I also managed it by building my skills and confidence.

As you work through this book, we will continue this journey together. I will guide you as you explore your test anxiety and provide you with everything you need to know to successfully manage it. Now, it's time to move on to Step 2 in this process.

## Step 2: What Are Your Symptoms of Test Anxiety?

The next step on your journey is about learning how your experiences with test anxiety and panic affect you. This process requires a bit of reflection on your past experiences, but it isn't complicated. You only need a journal or notes app, a pen or pencil, and 10 minutes. But why use journaling?

This activity has several benefits and is especially useful for managing stress and anxiety. It can also be fun to practice. The main thing to keep in mind when developing your own journaling practice is that no one is going to read what you write, so it doesn't have to be perfect. You can use slang and abbreviations, or simply write in a way that makes the most sense to you.

It's also important to remind yourself to be honest and write without judging yourself. The goal is to turn your thoughts into a physical form you can reflect on to not only alleviate stress and anxiety but also determine their cause. This makes it easier to figure out which coping mechanisms might help you, allowing you to take action in a way that's empowering and effective for you.

Before we work on identifying your anxiety symptoms, you need to first understand how to journal. There's no right or wrong way; however, there are a few methods you could choose from.

### *Method 1: Write About Your Concerns*

If you have specific concerns, like feeling anxious about an upcoming exam, you can write about it. State what you're worried about and explain why. Then, use the question "Why?" to help you dive deeper into your thoughts to identify their cause, whether you're worried about something else, and how these concerns may be affecting other areas of your life. Asking why three to five times will prompt effective introspection.

### *Method 2: Take Part in Freewriting*

This form of journaling allows you to simply write about whatever is on your mind during that moment without censoring your thoughts or editing them. Freewriting is valuable when you want to explore feelings and thought processes to gain a better understanding of what's going on inside your mind. To prevent this lack of topic boundaries from feeling overwhelming, consider setting a 10- or 15-minute timer for your first few journaling sessions.

### *Method 3: Make Use of Journaling Prompts*

It can be overwhelming to attempt to simply write whatever comes to your mind. You may even find that your mind goes blank as soon as you put your pen to paper, evoking memories of all the times you have frozen during a test, and that can put you off the idea of journaling. This is when prompts can become useful. They provide you with a starting point and give you a specific focus or problem to solve during your writing session. You can even revisit the same prompt multiple times.

Now, it's time to put these methods and the information from this chapter into action.

## *Activity 1*

1. Using the information from this chapter, write down the symptoms of anxiety that you have already experienced.
2. Reflect on the situations during which these symptoms manifested:
    a. What were you doing?
    b. How did you feel?
    c. Were you already stressed out by additional responsibilities or situations before entering the situation where these symptoms intensified?
3. Briefly describe whether you feel these symptoms only during testing and presentation situations or if you also experience them during other circumstances.

## *Activity 2*

1. Briefly describe your current concern. In terms of anxiety, this likely includes concerns about what *could* happen.
2. Consider why you think this scenario could happen using the following questions to guide you in understanding your concerns better by laying out the evidence:
    a. Who might be involved in the scenario?
    b. What could happen during this scenario?
    c. When might this event happen?
    d. Where could this scenario occur?
    e. Why do you think this scenario happened?

f. How did this scenario occur?

3. Lay out the possible events as steps so that you can understand what would happen **before** your concern occurs and what could happen **afterward**.

4. Explain what action you could take if the worst-case scenario does happen. (Take note that these actions could include strategies that will be discussed in future chapters.)

5. After completing the above steps, take a deep breath and reflect on your emotions:

    a. Compared to when you first started this activity, how do you feel about your concern?

    b. Are you as stressed out as you were originally, or do you feel like you're more prepared?

## Key Takeaways

In this chapter, we explored anxiety, including its causes, symptoms, and impact. You now understand that the physical and mental symptoms of anxiety can also be experienced when you have a panic attack. Being able to identify the symptoms you experience, as well as their effects, provides you with the opportunity to develop a targeted treatment plan and track your progress using the remainder of the steps in this book. We also learned that

- it's normal to experience anxiety when preparing for tests.
- anxiety becomes a problem when it starts to interfere with your ability to perform on the test.
- anxiety and panic can manifest in physical and psychological symptoms that are experienced at varying intensities.

- panic can make you believe that you're dying due to its intensity, but it doesn't mean you are at risk of dying.

From this chapter, you should also understand that your thoughts and beliefs play a very important role in test anxiety. In the next chapter, we're going to dive deeper into the impact that your mindset can have on test anxiety and how you can harness the power of your mind to benefit you instead.

## Chapter 3:

# The Role of Mindset

Learning to manage your test anxiety and overcome the obstacles that this type of anxiety creates doesn't require any fancy tools. In fact, you already have everything you need, and your mind is the most powerful tool that you possess.

As technology and science have developed, we've been able to study the brain in more detail to gain a better understanding of how it works and the impact its health and functioning can have on the rest of the body. Research on the connection between the mind and the body has provided us with valuable insight into the impact that mental health conditions, like anxiety and depression, may have on the rest of your well-being. But this connection is a two-way street, meaning that your physical health and conditions like gastrointestinal issues, for example, may impact your mental health as well.

The easiest way to think of the impact your mental state—which is affected by your test anxiety—can have on your body is to remember any moment where you felt nervous. This could have been during a test, before you went on a date, or when you met a new person. The feeling commonly described as "butterflies in the stomach" demonstrates how your emotions and thoughts can manifest in both your mind *and* your body. This information is valuable when learning to manage your test anxiety.

The previous chapter discussed several physical symptoms of test anxiety, further supporting the idea that your mental state can have a big impact on your physical health. It also tells us that the strategies you use to manage your test anxiety shouldn't solely focus on taking care of your mental well-being. Instead, your approach to managing your test anxiety should consider your overall well-being to ensure that the methods you use are truly effective.

This is where mindset comes into play. Mindset is sometimes dismissed as a useful tool because people believe that any substantial change will require them to only think positive thoughts. In reality, it's impossible to be positive about life all the time. Even people who appear to have a very positive mindset will have days where they feel sad or angry. It's important and healthy to allow yourself to feel all your emotions so that you can process them. The key is to not get stuck in them.

Unfortunately, negative emotions are very skilled at keeping their hold on your mental and emotional state. Learning to shift your mindset means developing the ability to identify, reflect on, process, and let go of your negative thoughts without getting stuck in them.

When you can do this, you'll find it easier to implement strategies that allow you to work through and manage your anxiety better. This includes learning to reframe your negative thoughts when they arise before and during testing situations so that your thoughts can serve you instead of harming you. We'll discuss these methods in detail in later chapters.

By shifting your mindset when you experience test anxiety, you can turn your thoughts into a tool that benefits you instead of hindering you. Let's start by investigating what the mind is capable of.

## The Power of the Mind

I like to study the work of Dr. Alia Crum and her colleagues at the Stanford Mind and Body Lab when learning about the power of mindset. Their work has provided evidence that supports the theory that the mind is a powerful role-player in our lives. Dr. Crum's work is especially valuable since she is not only an influential psychologist and assistant professor at Stanford University but is also known for her innovative research on the psychology of mindset and its impact on health and performance. Her research focuses on how changes in mindset may alter health outcomes, behaviors, and stress responses. Since we want to uncover the role of mindset in understanding and managing test anxiety, her work is a very valuable source of information.

This is also where the placebo effect needs to be considered. This effect is often seen as a nuisance by researchers who are trying to ensure accuracy and consistency in their studies, but it can actually provide valuable insight into the mind's ability to trigger beneficial physiological changes (Howe et al., 2022).

Dr. Crum and her colleagues have discovered that a person's expectations and beliefs about the treatment they are undergoing can significantly influence the outcome and resulting physiological changes of said treatment (Howe et al., 2022). This means that mindset—which takes the form of the placebo effect here—can influence the effectiveness of various medications and therapeutic treatments, so it could be vital to successfully managing a variety of mental and physical health conditions.

But I want us to specifically look at Dr. Crum's work on rethinking stress. Dr. Crum has introduced the concept of the "stress mindset." This is based on the idea that the way a person perceives stress can have a noticeable impact on their well-being. Studies suggest that if a person believes that stress is beneficial, they will experience better health and performance outcomes in comparison to a person who believes that stress is debilitating (Crum et al., 2023).

This idea is further supported by Dr. Crum's research on stress mindset interventions. Her work has demonstrated that even a brief intervention that helps to shift a person's perspective on stress can lead to better health and performance outcomes. In one study, participants who viewed stress as beneficial reported lower levels of anxiety and greater feelings of control and resilience. They also felt more capable of handling stress and using it to their advantage instead of being negatively affected by it (Crum et al., 2023).

So, what does this mean for us? Well, Dr. Crum's research supports the idea that shifting the way that you think about stress can actually lower your anxiety and benefit your well-being. This is exciting because it helps us understand that our minds have the power to change outcomes, making it a valuable tool in managing and overcoming test anxiety.

## *What Is Mindset?*

While the previous section gives us insight into what the mind is capable of, you're probably wondering how exactly it can benefit your journey to overcoming test anxiety. To truly understand the benefits you may experience, you have to understand what mindset is and how it works.

Mindset is often defined as the set of core beliefs you use to understand yourself and the world around you. These beliefs affect how you see yourself, your expectations, and how you interpret and understand other people and the world we live in, as well as how you approach goals and obstacles. As such, your mindset has the ability to shape the reality you live in.

Your mindset can't truly be "right" or "wrong;" however, it can still impact how you live your life and see yourself. This is also why no two people will have exactly the same mindset. Instead, we categorize mindsets into two main categories:

- **Fixed:** A fixed mindset is based on the belief that your abilities and traits are inherent and cannot be changed. This means that you may think that you can't achieve your academic goals because you weren't born with the talent to do complicated math equations, so why should you bother trying to put in the work to develop this skill?
- **Growth:** When you believe that skills and talents are developed through hard work and consistent effort, you are inspired to develop learning-oriented goals that allow you to see challenges and setbacks as opportunities. So, when you have a growth mindset and you struggle with your coursework, you see it as an opportunity to develop your knowledge and skills using tools like asking for help, working with a tutor, and attending study groups.

As you can see, mindset is about more than your thought patterns. It also includes your core beliefs and the physical actions you take to follow through on your thoughts. The good news is that regardless of your current mindset, you can shift it to one that serves you better, so it can be a valuable tool for managing test anxiety. But harnessing your mindset means knowing how it works.

## *The Inner Workings of Mindset*

Mindset is powerful because it can impact how you interpret the world. This means that the situations your mind and body prepare for and how you feel about yourself and your capabilities are affected too. If you have a negative mindset about taking tests due to your test anxiety, for example, then your mind and body will prepare for a negative experience and allow doubts about your skills and knowledge to take charge.

The key thing to remember about your mindset is that while its impact on you and your life is very real, your mindset may not be an accurate reflection of the reality you live in. Reflect on the example from the previous paragraph: Your test anxiety may contribute to doubts about your ability to succeed in your academics; however, this doesn't mean you aren't capable of succeeding. If you identify the areas where you struggle and seek help, you could improve your skills and knowledge to overcome the obstacles you're facing.

This is also the process you're following by working through this book. The steps we're discussing aim to help you overcome your test anxiety, but they're also helping you shift your mindset to one that's more adaptable and allows you to pursue success despite the challenges that you may face.

Understanding your current mindset gives you the information you need to shift it. This means that you can take back control by making conscious decisions that will benefit your mental and physical well-being, allowing you to manage your test anxiety and feel confident in your test-taking abilities. The best way to do this is to develop an adaptive mindset.

An adaptive mindset is a type of growth mindset that helps people face and overcome various challenges in their lives. It involves changing how you view your test anxiety and the stress that accompanies it. While it's easy to see your test anxiety as the enemy, adopting an adaptive mindset means acknowledging that high levels of test anxiety can be harmful, but when managed correctly, it can also have benefits.

Test anxiety can help improve your focus, ensure that you remain alert, and keep you motivated when you have to spend hours preparing for tests. If you can acknowledge test anxiety's positive traits and see it as a tool that could possibly benefit you, you not only take away some of its power but also decrease its negative impact on your mental and physical well-being.

Simply put, you're reframing your negative thoughts about test anxiety, including your test-taking abilities so that they are more positive. In this way, you cultivate inspiration and motivation that helps you continue pursuing your academic goals regardless of the challenges you face. But does reframing your thoughts about stress really work?

## *The Stress Mindset*

In addition to Dr. Crum's work—which we discussed at the start of this chapter—other researchers have also investigated the impact of mindset on stress. In this section, we'll take a closer look at the findings of these studies so that you can see that changing your mindset about your test anxiety really will benefit you.

You have to understand that when you experience stress, your body goes through changes so that it can respond appropriately to the stressor. The way you respond can depend on various factors that fall outside the scope of this book.

However, in general, different chemicals, like adrenaline and cortisol, are released in the body when you experience stress. Adrenaline is commonly associated with the fight-or-flight response, which we know is also a type of anxiety reaction. But cortisol, known as the "stress hormone," is also released when you experience a mental or physical stressor like test anxiety. This hormone is responsible for ensuring that your body is ready to take action and respond appropriately to the stressor. While a test or exam is not a physical threat, your body's cortisol levels may increase since your mind perceives the test or exam as potentially harmful to your well-being.

While experiencing high levels of stress hormones like cortisol over long periods can be harmful to your well-being, you may also experience higher levels of cortisol during situations and experiences you perceive as exciting and positive. This means that cortisol's role in the stress response could actually contribute to increasing your energy and lowering your fatigue (Hoyt et al., 2016). This is valuable for testing periods since it may help you stay alert, concentrate better, and have the energy needed to prepare for and complete the exam.

A study that aimed to better understand mindset's role on the impact of stress discovered that people who believe stress will negatively impact their well-being, and experience a high amount of stress, are more likely to die within the next eight years in comparison to the study's participants who experienced large amounts of stress but reported that they didn't believe that it had a large impact on their well-being (Keller et al., 2012).

This means that it may not be your test anxiety that's solely responsible for the challenges you face. It may be the combination of a negative mindset about your test anxiety and exams, in addition to high levels of anxiety, that's affecting how you approach test taking and preparation.

While no one can control everything in their life, there are various strategies you can use to help you adapt and cope with anxiety and stress in healthy ways. Shifting your mindset is an especially useful technique since it makes use of the mind's natural powers so that you can succeed and cope with unexpected challenges.

## Shifting Your Mindset

Now that you understand just how powerful your mind can be, as well as the importance of your mindset, you can move on to learning about the value of shifting your mindset. This strategy is crucial to helping you overcome your test anxiety and cope with stress more effectively.

To get started, you have to understand your current thought patterns by exploring who you believe you are as a student. These thoughts are called "core beliefs." Core beliefs are a strong set of beliefs that form the very essence of who you are as a person, thus laying the foundation for your mindset. They play a role in shaping how you perceive the world, yourself, and your abilities, and they influence your thought patterns and behaviors.

Exploring your core beliefs can be scary because you're essentially questioning the essence of your being; however, this activity is important for managing test anxiety. Take note that core beliefs are not always accurate or based on factual evidence either. That's because these beliefs are formed through our early life experiences and our interactions with the world and other people.

Our core beliefs have the power to affect how we interpret our abilities, interactions with other people, and the world around us. This affects how we react in different situations, like taking tests. Since core beliefs are powerful, when they are negative, they can put you at risk of being held back and prevented from pursuing your goals. But how do you know what your core beliefs are?

While you will have different core beliefs for different areas in your life, we'll focus on the impact of your academic core beliefs since they are the ones that mainly contribute to your test anxiety. Examine the following list of negative core beliefs related to poor academic performance, and note in your journal which beliefs you relate to or have thought of in the past:

- **"I am not smart enough:"** You believe that your intellectual capabilities are inherently limited.

- **"I can't do anything right:"** A general belief that any attempt you make to improve your academics will only result in mistakes and failure.

- **"Professors don't like me:"** A belief that your educators are biased against you, resulting in unfair treatment and preventing you from pursuing support.

- **"I don't belong here:"** When you feel out of place or like you don't fit in academically. This belief often arises when you're in an academically competitive environment. It is also common in first-generation university students who don't have family knowledge of third-level education requirements to fall back on.

- **"I am a failure:"** This general self-assessment causes you to label yourself as inadequate or unsuccessful in your academic pursuits before you even get started.

- **"Other students are smarter than me:"** Thinking your peers are more capable and intelligent than you are makes you believe that you are inferior in comparison.

- **"I am not good at this subject:"** You specifically believe that you lack the ability to perform well in a specific academic area, like physics or math.

- **"No one can help me:"** You believe that it's pointless to seek out help because no one will understand or be able to provide you with the right guidance.

- **"Success is only for the lucky and privileged:"** The belief that academic success is determined by factors out of your control, like your socioeconomic status and luck.

- **"The educational system is unfair, and I can never get ahead:"** A belief that external factors, like a biased grading or unfair system, are responsible for poor academic outcomes.

- **"It doesn't matter how hard I try:"** You may experience feelings of helplessness and futility stemming from a belief that no matter how much effort you put in, the outcome will not change.

You may feel anxious as you read through the above list, but you don't have anything to be ashamed of. Remember that these beliefs aren't an accurate reflection of reality, but recognizing and reflecting on your negative core beliefs is key to helping you break free from their hold.

One of my negative core beliefs about academics that I always struggled with was believing that everyone else was smarter than me. I only developed this belief during my first year of college because it was truly the first time in my life that I had struggled with academics. While it wasn't true, this core belief held me back and severely impacted how I perceived myself and my abilities, further contributing to my test anxiety.

It was jarring too. I went from an academic environment I was familiar with and comfortable in to suddenly being amongst the best and brightest students from across the country. Of course, I wouldn't be the smartest student there, but that didn't mean I wasn't smart at all. This deeply ingrained negative belief took years of significant cognitive work for me to unlearn, but it was worth it because changing my thoughts was one of the most important things I had to do to achieve success. And you can do it too! First, let's take a closer look at the relationship between your limiting beliefs and test anxiety.

## *The Role of Limiting Beliefs*

Negative thoughts are always put in a bad light because they can contribute to problems like increased anxiety, feelings of unworthiness, low self-esteem, depression, fear, panic attacks, and stress. But the truth is that it's normal to experience negative thoughts. Problems arise when these thoughts are ongoing and persistent, making it difficult for you to move out of the negative headspace they have caused.

What's interesting is that we actually have the built-in ability to notice our negative thoughts. It's a skill that originates from ancestors who had to survive in harsh conditions, surrounded by threats to their survival. Negative thoughts in this context acted as a warning that signaled they were in danger. Being able to identify these thoughts quickly ensured that they were able to respond appropriately so that they could continue to survive.

This is known as "negativity bias," and it essentially means that your mind will notice negative thoughts, experiences, and comments more easily than positive ones. Negativity bias can make it challenging to see the good in everyday life since your mind is prioritizing anything it perceives to be negative.

For example, you may initially think that you had a bad day. Yet, upon reflection, you can recognize that you simply had one moment where you spilled your cup of coffee or forgot your textbook at home, while the rest of the day was enjoyable because your friend surprised you with a new notebook and your professor congratulated you on an assignment.

Negativity bias means that you're at a higher risk of holding on to negative experiences, like that time you got a low mark despite all the hard work you put into preparing for an exam. This makes it challenging to focus on the good in your life, and it could further fuel your test anxiety. These subconscious roadblocks can also stop you from pursuing your dreams by keeping you in your comfort zone, thereby affecting more than your academic life. Growth becomes almost impossible too since the resulting negative mindset will lead to increased anxiety, imposter syndrome, and procrastination.

Succumbing to negativity bias causes your inner voice to become more negative and critical, eventually causing the thoughts that arise in your mind during the day to become more negative. Limiting beliefs, also called "automatic negative thoughts" (ANTs), will continue to rise if you have a negative mindset. You may not even realize that your thoughts are always negative or that they're impacting your academics and mental well-being.

These ANTs originate from the negative core beliefs that are responsible for forming a negative mindset. This means that learning to identify your negative core beliefs allows you to take the first step to overcoming them, which we will discuss in later chapters. When you can identify your ANTs and your negative core beliefs, you can work toward developing a healthier and more adaptive way of interacting with the world. This allows you to manage your test anxiety effectively and approach any test with a more positive and adaptive mindset.

## Step 3: Acknowledging Your Limiting Beliefs

Now that you know what negative core beliefs are, you need to identify *your* core beliefs. This is crucial to helping you overcome them and shift your mindset in a way that helps you manage and overcome your test anxiety effectively.

In the section *Shifting Your Mindset*, you were provided with a list of negative core beliefs. I want you to reflect on the core beliefs that you related to before answering the questions that follow in your journal or notes app:

1. Consider how your family talks about intelligence. Write down how they would define intelligence.

2. Take a moment to think about intelligence, and write down your own definition, using what you believe intelligence is.

3. How does your definition differ from your family's definition of intelligence?

4. What do you think makes a person successful?

5. Are you seen as the smart family member? In childhood, what comments were made by your family about your capabilities?

6. Describe your earliest memory of school or the earliest academic experience you can remember.

    a. Was this experience positive or negative?

    b. Did you walk away from this experience with new beliefs about yourself or your abilities that you didn't have before?

7. Were you seen as smart by your teachers?

8. When reflecting on your interactions with peers and classmates, were you considered the smart one or was this title given to someone else?

If you weren't considered a smart student, take a moment to reflect on how this perception made you feel and write these emotions down.

9. Reflect on your answers to the above and the list of negative core beliefs from earlier, and create a new list of core beliefs you've identified using this reflection on your experiences and perceptions.

## Key Takeaways

In this chapter, we began exploring the power of our minds and thoughts. This is a key concept in cognitive behavioral therapy since our thoughts have the power to influence our feelings and actions—a concept that has been supported by Dr. Crum's research. But this doesn't mean we are powerless.

You already have everything you need to change your thoughts. This involves learning to identify and acknowledge negative thoughts and their impact, even though this activity can be uncomfortable. So, what are some other takeaways from this chapter?

- Core beliefs are the strong set of beliefs that make up the very essence of who you are as a person.
- These beliefs can shape how you perceive the world, your thought patterns, and your behaviors.
- Negative thoughts stem from negative core beliefs and can have a significantly harmful impact on your life and well-being.
- Negative core beliefs form a negative mindset, and by reframing your core beliefs to ones that are more beneficial and positive, you can shift your mindset to one that is adaptable.

- Learning to shift the way you think can help you improve your mental health and manage your test anxiety.

We covered a lot of technical information in this chapter, but it has given you the starting point for shifting your mindset. It's now time to investigate how you can change your core beliefs in a way that helps you manage your test anxiety.

## Chapter 4:

# Let's Change Your Mind

Identifying your negative beliefs and how they shape your mindset creates the foundation needed for successfully combating your negative thoughts. This allows you to turn limiting beliefs that would otherwise hinder you into positive thoughts that serve you and help you meet your goals. And this skill is especially valuable when navigating test anxiety and its management.

As you work through this chapter, reflect on what you learned from the previous chapter and keep the activities you completed close by. You will need this information to help you complete the exercises discussed here. Again, you don't need any special tools, just your journal or notes app. Your mind is powerful, and putting your thoughts into writing makes it easier for you to evaluate and reflect on them, helping you to make connections and implement beneficial methods for combating negative thoughts.

Before we dive into these different strategies, you first have to understand how your negative core beliefs have been affecting you, your academic career, and your goals.

## The Impact of Negative Core Beliefs

You have to keep in mind that your negative core beliefs will lead to the manifestation of limiting thoughts. As we discovered in the previous chapter, Dr. Crum's work demonstrates that these beliefs can have a big impact on your well-being and how you approach life—including how you prepare for tests and exams. This means that understanding your negative core beliefs and how they impact you is crucial to helping you manage your test anxiety.

Think of it like purposefully studying the strengths and weaknesses of your enemy (test anxiety) to create an effective battle plan. Using this information, you can choose strategies that will help you meet the needs you identified and make it easier to tailor any strategies you use to suit your specific circumstances and experiences. This ensures the effectiveness of the methods you implement and can help you shift your mindset and feel more confident about overcoming your negative core beliefs.

To create an effective battle plan, you have to build on the information from the previous chapter. In this section, we're going to look at how your negative core beliefs may be affecting you and contributing to your test anxiety.

### *Avoidance*

When you feel very stressed out or anxious, you might try to avoid the cause of your fears. After all, if you avoid the trigger of these upsetting feelings, you aren't forced to deal with the uncomfortable and negative emotions or thoughts that accompany the challenging situation. Unfortunately, this unhealthy coping mechanism can do a lot of harm.

Avoidance often manifests when you believe that you're bad at a challenging task or subject or when you aren't immediately good at something, like a new skill. With test anxiety, this can lead to gaps in your knowledge and skills that could cause problems later in your academic career or life. And the simple act of thinking you can't do something fuels this behavior even further, widening this gap and creating a negative feedback loop. That's pretty scary!

Incomplete homework or avoiding going to specific classes because you think to yourself, *What's the point if I'm not going to learn anything anyway?* are just two examples of what avoidance might look like for you.

### *Increased Procrastination*

Procrastination is often viewed as being "lazy," but it rarely results from simply not wanting to do the activity in question. You may be afraid, or the task may trigger uncomfortable emotions, leading to procrastination—a specific form of avoidance. Even the most organized and well-prepared individuals put off and delay tasks that they don't enjoy, that trigger feelings of anxiety and stress, or that are challenging. So, procrastination is pretty common.

In the case of test anxiety, procrastination may look like putting off preparing for upcoming tests or only completing an assignment at the last minute. While you will probably eventually deal with the thing you are avoiding, it can still lead to negative emotions and consequences like poor performance. Other examples include waiting until it's too late to attend your professor's office hours to ask questions about the upcoming assignment or putting off going to study groups.

## *Low Motivation and Perfectionism*

When you lack the motivation to do a task, like working on that upcoming assignment, you may put it off, causing you to procrastinate. A lack of motivation could also arise when you're afraid that you won't be able to complete the assignment without making mistakes. And if you won't get it right the first time, or it won't be perfect, why bother? Does this sound familiar?

But there is more to this than simply being a perfectionist or fearing that the outcome won't meet your expectations. A belief that you're inadequate can contribute to a lack of *intrinsic motivation* to engage with your academic materials. Intrinsic motivation is important because it doesn't rely on external rewards. Instead, it occurs because the act of working on the activity provides you with a sense of satisfaction.

A lack of intrinsic motivation sets you up for failure anyway because external motivation and willpower are limited resources that will inevitably leave you wanting when you need to put long-term effort into seeking success. By unintentionally setting yourself up for failure, you reinforce the negative core beliefs that led you here.

### *Self-Sabotaging Behaviors*

Self-sabotage can be a conscious or unconscious behavior that prevents you from achieving your goals. The behaviors you engage in during self-sabotage are harmful behaviors that can result in negative consequences like failure. When you engage in self-sabotaging behaviors, you're reinforcing your negative core beliefs, causing you to unintentionally continue limiting yourself.

### *Increased Anxiety and Stress*

While feeling anxious about an upcoming test is normal, your anxiety may become heightened when you struggle with persistent negative beliefs about your academic performance. Your anxiety may become even worse when you're struggling with the manifestations of these beliefs like procrastination, avoidance, low motivation, and self-sabotaging behaviors.

Eventually, these high levels of stress and anxiety may cause physical symptoms that further affect how you feel about yourself and your ability to prepare for and complete the test or exam.

As you can see, the impact of your negative core beliefs can be extremely damaging. That's why it's crucial that you take these beliefs seriously and work to change them. Keep the list of negative core beliefs you identified in the previous chapter close by, and work through the introspective prompts below so that you can start making connections between these beliefs and how they've supported your test anxiety.

### *Reflection Activity*

After reading through the impacts that negative core beliefs can have, you can begin to understand how your own core beliefs have impacted you. This means you are going to identify how you've been impacted by your negative core beliefs. You can use the following guidelines to help you:

This reflection activity will help you start the process of understanding how you have been affected by your negative core beliefs. But we don't want to get stuck in this negativity, so how do you change your mind?

## Strategies for Changing Your Mind

In the last chapter, we identified your limiting beliefs. Now, it's time to change these beliefs into thoughts that are realistic, positive, and beneficial. While there are many strategies you could choose from, we're going to take a look at cognitive restructuring techniques, as they are both accessible and incredibly effective.

Cognitive restructuring is a tool within cognitive behavioral therapy that helps you identify and challenge your negative thought patterns—which we know influence your core beliefs and mindset—so that you can begin changing them to realistic and positive thoughts that will serve you.

Keep in mind that the goal of this method is to help you achieve a thinking pattern that is realistic and balanced. You're examining a negative thought, understanding it, acknowledging why it may have arisen, and then implementing strategies that help you shift this thought to one that serves you better. This more realistic affirmation is then reinforced using your actions and words.

While cognitive restructuring isn't made up of specific steps, the following techniques have been designed to help you alter your way of thinking. These methods are especially valuable since you can easily tailor them to your unique needs and the challenges you experience.

## *Socratic Questioning*

This technique is a type of communication style that aims to stimulate critical thinking using open-ended questions. Such questions help you become more aware of your thoughts, feelings, and behaviors, making it easier to understand why they may arise and when.

Simply put, having the ability to examine the validity and logic of your thoughts and beliefs allows you to analyze the evidence that supports or challenges a specific belief, like a negative belief about your academic abilities, giving you the power to change your mind.

This method requires a step-by-step approach. We'll work through the following example to help you get a better idea of how this method works.

**Negative thought:** *My professor doesn't like me, so I'm not going to get a good grade in this class.*

1. **Clarifying the statement**
    - **Question:** What specific actions or behaviors from your professor make you think that they don't like you?
        - **Purpose:** To encourage you to gather detailed and concrete evidence that led to the creation of this belief.
2. **Probing the assumptions**
    - **Question:** What assumptions are you making about your professor's actions or words?
        - **Purpose:** To help you identify any underlying assumptions you may be making, as these assumptions may or may not be accurate.
3. **Exploring the evidence and reasons**

- **Question:** Can you provide specific examples of when you felt your professor acted in a way that indicated they do not like you?
    - **Purpose:** The goal is to identify specific moments or interactions instead of just your feelings.
- **Question:** How has your professor behaved toward other students in situations similar to the ones you identified?
    - **Purpose:** To determine how your professor treats you in comparison to your peers.
- **Question:** Has your professor ever provided you with feedback or comments that indicate that they don't like you?
    - **Purpose:** To identify evidence to support or deny the original statement by examining your professor's words and actions toward you.

4. **Looking for and studying alternative explanations**

- **Question:** Are there other potential reasons for your professor's behavior that don't involve them disliking you?
    - **Purpose:** To identify alternative explanations for your professor's behavior.
- **Question:** Could your professor's behavior be a result of factors that are unrelated to you, like the stressors they're experiencing outside of class or their teaching style?
    - **Purpose:** To explore external factors that are unrelated to you and which may be influencing your professor's behavior.

5. **Probing the implication and consequences**

    - **Question:** How does the belief that your professor doesn't like you affect your performance and attitude in class and when working on the coursework for this class?
        - **Purpose:** To understand how this belief affects you.
    - **Question:** If you believed that your professor felt neutrally or supportive toward you, what would change?
        - **Purpose:** To explore how a different belief can influence how you approach the class, its coursework, and tests.

6. **Question the question**

    - **Question:** Why is it so important to you to figure out whether your professor likes you or not? How has this belief affected your academic goals?
        - **Purpose:** To challenge the importance of the belief in relation to your academic success.
    - **Question:** What would happen if you focused on your own performance instead of giving so much attention to your professor's perceived feelings about you?
        - **Purpose:** To shift your focus toward factors you actually have control over.

As you can see, there are many questions you could use to help you analyze your negative beliefs and thoughts. The questions discussed above form part of a process that's specifically designed to help you thoroughly evaluate whether or not there is enough evidence to support the negative thought. Let's take a look at how this kind of Socratic question could play out in a conversation with your therapist:

You: "I think my professor doesn't like me."

Dr. Busch: "What makes you think that? Can you provide me with specific examples?"

You: "Well, during the last class we had, I raised my hand to answer a question she'd posed, but she didn't call on me."

Dr. Busch: "How often has this happened? Is it possible she didn't see you, or was there another reason?"

You: "It's happened a few times, but she might have been busy or didn't see me."

Dr. Busch: "How does she treat the other students in your class? Have you noticed her missing other students' raised hands?"

You: "Yes, sometimes she doesn't call on the other students either. Maybe, it's just her teaching style."

Dr. Busch: "Have you received any direct feedback from your professor that suggests she doesn't like you?"

You: "No, not directly. She actually gave me really positive feedback on my last assignment."

Dr. Busch: "So, the evidence suggests that your professor has been positive about your work. Could there be other reasons for her behavior in class?"

You: "Maybe, she's just trying to manage a busy lecture hall and sometimes misses hands."

Dr. Busch: "How do you think believing your professor doesn't like you affects your performance in class?"

You: "It makes me nervous and less likely to participate."

Dr. Busch: "What if you assumed that your professor felt neutral or positively toward you? How would that change your approach?"

You: "I'd probably feel more confident and participate in class more."

The majority of the time I complete this exercise with my patients, there is insufficient evidence to support their negative thoughts. This supports the idea that your negative thoughts aren't always an accurate reflection of your reality, so don't hesitate to question them. This will empower you to take action in a way that will benefit you instead.

***Reflection Activity***

In your journal or notes app, write down one negative thought or one of your core beliefs from the previous chapter's activity, and begin investigating it using the six Socratic questions from this section.

## *Reframing*

We've briefly touched upon reframing negative thoughts in previous chapters. This cognitive behavioral technique is valuable since it helps you shift your mindset so that you can alter your behavioral and emotional responses to a particular situation. This allows your perception and understanding of the situation to also shift, giving you the opportunity to learn and grow. So, what is reframing?

Open up your phone's camera, and point it at your textbook or a glass of water. If you move your phone closer to the object or further away, the frame through which you view it changes. You could also move around the object and view it from behind.

Reframing works the same way. You're examining your negative thoughts through a mental camera lens and shifting your perspective on the circumstances at hand. Instead of viewing them from one angle (in a negative way), you're changing your mental focus so that you can view these thoughts and their stimuli from a different angle, one that is more positive and constructive.

Let's take a look at how reframing may be performed by studying the two examples that follow.

*Example 1*

**Negative thought:** *It takes me forever to finish my problem sets.*

**Positive reframe:** *I take the time I need to understand and complete my problem sets thoroughly, and I'm working on strategies to improve my efficiency.*

While the original, negative thought might not seem like it could have a big impact, let's take a look at the different ways it could be affecting you:

- **Negative self-perception:** The negative thought is a type of negative self-assessment that suggests that you are slow or inefficient. This can hurt your self-esteem and contribute to a mindset that focuses on perceived inadequacies about your capabilities instead of your strengths.

- **Increased stress and anxiety levels:** When you believe that tasks will take long periods to complete—especially when you have to complete these same activities in timed exams—you may become more anxious and stressed out when working on them. This can make it challenging to stay focused and perform well, leading to even poorer progress that creates a repeating negative cycle.

- **Avoidance and procrastination:** Believing that an activity, like completing your problem sets, is going to take a long time can make you more likely to procrastinate working on them or developing the skills needed to complete them properly. This can result in rushed and low-quality work that negatively affects your overall grade and prevents you from truly understanding the material.

- **Fixed mindset:** The original, negative statement is an example of a fixed mindset, which we now know would prevent you from seeking out or using strategies that could help you develop your skills, improve your efficiency, and benefit your performance.

- **Lower motivation and engagement:** When you view problem sets as tasks that "take forever," you feel less motivated or interested in working on them. This could lead to additional feelings of overwhelm, making you less likely to put in the necessary effort, resulting in poorer outcomes.

How does the positive reframe affect you, then?

- **Positive self-perception:** When you acknowledge the effort it takes to understand the material thoroughly, you can boost your self-esteem and promote a mindset that focuses on learning and improvement.

- **Reduced stress and anxiety:** By framing the time you take to work on the problem set as necessary for properly understanding the work, you can decrease your stress and anxiety. This helps you feel calmer and can lead to a more effective and self-compassionate approach to problem sets in the future.

- **Increased productivity:** The reframed statement emphasizes the additional work you're putting in to improve your efficiency. This encourages proactive behavior that can help you find study methods that are more effective and help you manage your time better.

- **Growth mindset:** This mindset is encouraged when using the positive reframe since it helps you believe in your ability to improve over time. A growth mindset is valuable, as it helps you stay motivated, seek help, and improve and practice your skills.

- **Enhanced motivation and engagement:** By purposefully recognizing the value of taking time to understand your problem sets properly, you can increase your motivation and engagement with the work. This helps you feel more invested in your coursework and the learning process, resulting in an overall better performance and academic success.

*Example 2*

**Negative thought:** *I failed my exam, so that must mean I'm stupid.*

**Positive reframe:** *I didn't perform well on this exam, but it is an opportunity for me to identify where I need to improve so that I can develop better study strategies and identify areas where I need to ask for help.*

It's easy to see that the negative thought will only harm you and your progress. Let's take a look at how you may be impacted:

- **Negative self-concept:** Labeling yourself as "stupid" after a single test damages your self-esteem and creates a fixed perception that hinders you. This means that your future academic efforts will be negatively impacted by this belief that you are not smart or capable.

- **Fixed mindset:** This original, negative thought contributes to a fixed mindset that encourages you to believe that intelligence is something that is unchangeable. It can prevent you from making any effort to develop your knowledge and skills and may lead you to believe that any effort you put in is a waste of time. When you encounter setbacks and challenges, you won't try to overcome them either.

- **Increased anxiety and stress:** When you equate failure with a lack of intelligence, you can increase your stress and anxiety levels. The negative emotions that arise will cause further damage to your ability to concentrate, learn, and perform on future tests and academic tasks.

- **Avoidance of challenges:** Believing that you are inherently incapable of succeeding on the exam can lead you to avoid challenging tasks and subjects in the future. This may lead to you missing out on valuable opportunities that would allow you to grow and develop your skills, causing you to experience further academic difficulties due to gaps in your knowledge and skills.

- **Decreased motivation:** Your motivation to put in work for the subject you did poorly in may decrease significantly when you believe that you are stupid. This can lead you to think that any effort you put in would be pointless and thus contribute to a lack of engagement with your coursework, resulting in even poorer academic outcomes that only reinforce the negative thought.

It's crucial that you understand how your positive reframe benefits and empowers you:

- **Positive self-concept:** Being able to recognize that poor performance on an exam is a reflection of the specific challenges you faced, and not your overall intelligence, can help you maintain a positive self-image. This is crucial for developing resilience so that you can continue to try regardless of the outcome.

- **Growth mindset:** This mindset is promoted when you use the positive reframe to combat negative thoughts. That's because the reframed statement allows you to view your abilities as improvable if you put in the effort and are willing to learn new things. You will then begin to view challenges as opportunities for growth instead of threats to your self-worth.

- **Reduced anxiety and stress:** Purposefully perceiving your exam results as an opportunity for you to learn, instead of evidence of your intelligence (or lack thereof), can help you decrease your anxiety and stress levels. This fosters a healthier and more productive approach to learning.

- **Embracing challenges:** Embracing challenges and persisting in the face of setbacks and obstacles becomes easier when you believe that you can improve your intelligence, abilities, and skills. This makes it easier to put in the work to learn and develop your skills, even if it takes time.

- **Increased motivation and engagement:** By taking the time to recognize and understand that effort and hard work can lead to improvement, you can increase your motivation to try. It also becomes easier to take the time to prepare, seek out help, and pursue more useful strategies that will help you improve your performance.

***Reflection Activity***

Take one of your negative thoughts, and write it down in your journal or notes app. Then, use the following instructions:

1. Ask yourself how you can reframe this thought so that it's more positive.
2. Take a moment to reflect on the new statement and identify
    a. the positive feelings that arise.
    b. the thoughts it inspires.
    c. the actions it makes you want to take.

## *Affirmations*

You've probably heard about affirmations before, but what are they? Simply put, affirmations are clear statements that are positive and to the point. When you repeat them to yourself, you can combat negative and unhelpful thoughts and build your confidence in your abilities. They are useful for helping you shift your mindset and pursue your goals.

Affirmations are effective because they harness the power and adaptive nature of the mind. This has led to psychologists like David Sherman and Geoffrey Cohen studying their role in combating conditions like stress and anxiety. Sherman and Cohen (2014) have conducted research that specifically aims to understand the impact that self-affirmations can have in acting as a buffer against stress and promoting adaptive coping.

In their comprehensive review, they discovered that self-affirmations have the potential to help a person maintain their self-integrity, lower their need for defensiveness, and achieve more positive outcomes even after facing threats against their self-worth (Cohen & Sherman, 2014). So, how does this help you when you struggle with test anxiety?

A study conducted in 2016 by Borman, Grigg, and Hanselman aimed to investigate the effectiveness of self-affirmation interventions in reducing performance disparities between different student groups, with a focus on minority students. The study required students to complete exercises that would help them identify their core values and understand why they were important to them—similar to what we've been discussing. This exercise was repeated several times throughout the school year and included self-affirmation activities (Borman et al., 2016).

In addition to tracking participation in these exercises, the researchers collected the participating students' academic performance data to understand the impact that this intervention had on their academic achievements. The study found that self-affirmation interventions had a significantly positive impact on academic performance and confirmed that self-affirmations have the potential to narrow the achievement gap between minority students and their nonminority peers (Borman et al., 2016).

That's pretty incredible since self-affirmation isn't a complicated activity and doesn't require any special tools. As such, it's highly accessible, and you can also benefit from it.

When affirmations are used correctly, you can experience benefits like improved self-confidence and self-worth, helping you boost your overall self-esteem. Your thought patterns will also begin to shift and become more positive and beneficial, helping you develop a more optimistic outlook. Additionally, affirmations can reinforce any existing positive beliefs, helping you become more motivated and persistent in pursuing and achieving your goals.

In terms of test anxiety, affirmations can lower your stress and anxiety levels. This means you'll experience increased feelings of calm, and your mind will feel more focused. By developing a belief and confidence in your abilities through affirmations, you can improve your performance in various areas of your life, including your work, academics, and personal endeavors.

### *The Anatomy of Effective Self-Affirmations*

Personal affirmations aren't complicated to create, but they do require you to follow specific guidelines to ensure that they are effective. These guidelines can be used to help you create your own positive self-affirmations.

Self-affirmations must be

- **positive:** Your affirmations must always be stated positively to promote a constructive mindset. For instance, rather than stating, "I don't doubt myself," try "I believe in myself."

- **in the present tense:** Write your positive statement as if you have already achieved this state. This promotes your belief in your ability to achieve this state. For example, "I am improving my academic skills every day" will be more effective than "I will improve my academic skills."

- **personal:** The statement is unique to you and about you, so use "I" and "My" statements.

- **specific:** Be as clear and specific as possible when creating your affirmations so that they encourage you to focus on the particular goals or areas of improvement that you're trying to achieve.

- **believable:** While you want your statements to be positive, they should also be realistic and believable so that you can set yourself up for success when working toward goals and developing skills.

These principles provide you with a great starting point. So, what could your positive self-affirmations look like when you're trying to combat negative thoughts specifically?

- **Negative thought:** *I can't do this.*
    - **Positive affirmation:** "I am confident and capable in my abilities."
- **Negative thought:** *College is too hard for me.*
    - Positive affirmation: "I handle challenges with grace and resilience."
- **Negative thought:** *No one is giving me a chance.*
    - **Positive affirmation:** "I am worthy of opportunities, and my skills and efforts are being recognized by others."
- **Negative thought:** *I will never make it to law school.*
    - **Positive affirmation:** "Every opportunity I seek brings me one step closer to my success, and I am fully capable of creating my own chances."

*Reflection Activity*

Complete the following exercise in your journal or notes app:

1. Choose to either address the same negative thought from the previous activities or identify a new one.
2. Use the guidelines from this section to help you create a positive self-affirmation to challenge and counteract your chosen negative thought.

## Step 4: Challenge Your Negative Core Beliefs By Changing Your Mind

The previous section provided you with the exact methods you need to use to help you shift your mindset and overcome your negative core beliefs. Here, we'll quickly recap these methods and why they will benefit you. Feel free to come back to this section for some motivation any time you feel overwhelmed by negative thinking.

### *Method 1: Question the Negative Thought*

The goal of Socratic questioning is to help you assess the validity of negative and unhelpful thoughts. This allows you to determine if there's sufficient evidence to support the thought so that you can take appropriate action. Engaging with this method will empower you to develop a more helpful and positive way of thinking about the situation while implementing positive actions that support and reinforce your new positive thoughts.

### *Method 2: Reframe It*

It really can be helpful to view your thoughts or situation in a different way. Not only does this allow you to develop critical thinking skills and consider all the possibilities, but it also helps you develop a healthier and more balanced mindset that prompts you to continue pursuing your goals. You may even find it easier to overcome obstacles in the future after developing this skill.

### *Method 3: Use Positive Affirmations*

Positive statements have a lot more power than you may think. If you're a visual person, you can write your positive affirmations on paper cards—or even decorate these cards to make them appealing—and stick them on your mirror, in your textbooks, or in any area where you will see them. This helps you reinforce your new way of thinking, as you're able to read through your affirmations several times a day.

## Key Takeaways

In this chapter, we've reinforced the idea that negative core beliefs lead to negative thoughts that can harm your mental well-being and contribute to your test anxiety. Avoidance, procrastination, low motivation, anxiety, stress, and self-sabotage are just a few of the most harmful effects that negative thought patterns may trigger.

Through the use of the therapeutic process known as *cognitive restructuring*, you can counteract your negative thought patterns and shift your mindset to one that serves you instead of hindering you. This makes it easier for you to change your actions and feelings accordingly.

While the skills and techniques from this chapter and the previous one are crucial to combating test anxiety, you may still experience nervousness or uncertainty before and during tests. It's now time for us to discover how you can calm your mind and body using healthy coping mechanisms.

## Chapter 5:

# Learning to Relax on Purpose

From your own experiences with test anxiety, you're well aware that it can be a full-body experience. So, the strategies you use to manage and overcome your anxiety need to be able to calm both your mind and your body.

As daunting as this may be at first, you can find comfort in the fact that we've already covered some of the techniques that will help you care for your mental well-being when your test anxiety is triggered. These methods are also great for managing other forms of anxiety or any overwhelming emotions.

Now, it's time for us to dive into the strategies that will help you manage the physical effects of stress and anxiety so that you can continue strengthening your resilience and increasing your opportunities for academic success.

The techniques discussed in this chapter are healthy coping skills. They consist of thoughts and behaviors you can practice using specific steps to help you manage internal and external stressors. Coping skills can be practiced during any situation that causes you to feel stressed and anxious, like before and during an exam, when you are called upon during a lecture, or before you receive the results of a recent test.

Breathing exercises, mindfulness meditation, positive self-talk, journaling, engaging in hobbies or physical activity, seeking social support, and problem-solving techniques are just a few examples of healthy coping strategies that will benefit you when managing your test anxiety. You may even recognize some of these strategies from previous chapters.

Practicing these skills during situations that trigger your test anxiety is the best way to figure out which method may be more effective during a specific situation. For example, deep breathing could be more useful before a test, whereas grounding might be more helpful to you during the exam. By experimenting with these skills during different situations, you can determine which method, or combination of strategies, works best for you during a specific situation.

However, once you have discovered the coping mechanisms that work best for you, it is important to practice those techniques in non-stressful situations too. This will allow you to become familiar with using the skills, making it easier to use them when your anxiety arises. In the next section, we'll look at how coping mechanisms can benefit you, as well as how you can implement them in daily life.

## The Importance of Healthy Coping Skills

Coping skills are something that we develop from an early age without even realizing it. They help us tolerate, manage, and overcome challenging and uncomfortable situations. The problem is that the way you adapt to these situations can be negative or positive depending on the type of coping skills you've developed.

Harmful coping skills are exactly that, coping mechanisms that can cause short-term or long-term harm while helping you deal with the challenging situation. They can cause problems in your personal, academic, and professional life and may even end up harming your overall health.

Avoidance and procrastination are two potentially harmful coping mechanisms that you may use to survive your negative core beliefs. Substance abuse, like smoking or excessive alcohol intake, is another example of a negative coping skill you may use to manage intense feelings of anxiety.

Healthy coping mechanisms, on the other hand, allow you to cope with, manage, and overcome challenging situations in ways that benefit your overall well-being and provide room for growth. These skills also offer safer outlets for your anxious energy by providing you with constructive and positive activities like grounding, deep breathing, and physical movement.

When you struggle with test anxiety, developing healthy coping skills is crucial for promoting and maintaining the well-being of your mental and physical health. They can be incorporated into your daily routine and practiced when a stressful situation arises.

You could even think of healthy coping mechanisms as a type of on-the-go self-care since they help you become more in tune with your body and its needs. The positive impact they have can help you show up fully in all areas of your academics, empowering you to pursue and achieve success.

There are many coping techniques you could choose from, but our focus will be on breathing, grounding, and visualization. If you're a swimmer, singer, or yogi you may already be familiar with controlling your breathing and using it to help you move through difficult physical sensations.

If you're an athlete, you've also likely used practices like visualization to help you imagine a successful play. This is a technique I've used myself, even before I struggled with test anxiety. As a high school basketball player, I would visualize my free throws gracefully flowing through the net, which helped me to feel in control on the court. So, as you can see, the techniques we will discuss in this chapter have many applications, and whether they are new to you or they simply take on a different iteration of one you've already practiced, mastering these skills can increase your resilience and confidence, helping you to mitigate both the psychological and physiological manifestations of test anxiety.

Let's get started with the one tool you always have on hand: your breath.

## *Using Your Breath*

Breathing isn't an activity we consciously think about since it's an automatic bodily function. You also probably already know that this activity is vital because the movement of air in and out of your lungs allows for carbon dioxide to be expelled and oxygen to be absorbed, thereby ensuring your body can function properly. But did you know that the rate at which you breathe can impact your state of mind?

When you take short, shallow breaths, resulting in a rapid breathing pattern, you're more likely to feel anxious and on edge, whereas taking slow, deep breaths encourages a more relaxed and calmer state of mind. You can use this information to your advantage when managing your test anxiety. First, it's helpful to understand why this works.

Slow, deliberate breaths cause your diaphragm—the sheet of muscle located just underneath your ribs—to engage properly, allowing your body to inhale and exhale more air. This promotes relaxation and calms your nervous system. As an automatic function, breathing is regulated by the autonomic nervous system (ANS) which is further split into two systems: the parasympathetic nervous system (PNS) and the sympathetic nervous system (SNS).

The SNS is responsible for controlling your fight-or-flight response. Your PNS, on the other hand, is responsible for bringing your body back to a state of calm and rest, also known as the "rest-and-digest" state. So, these two systems balance each other out.

When your test anxiety has been triggered, your SNS will take charge. But you need to be able to calm down so that you can give the exam your full attention. This means that you need to learn to activate the PNS, which can be done by intentionally taking slow and deliberate breaths.

Deep breathing stimulates your vagus nerve. As the main nerve of your PNS, it's responsible for controlling bodily functions like heart rate, digestion, and your immune system. When activated, this nerve can promote relaxation, reduce your blood pressure, and lower your heart rate, helping you counteract the physiological effects of stress.

From previous chapters, we also learned that stress affects hormone levels. Your levels of the stress hormone, cortisol, will often rise when you become anxious. Deep breathing and slow exhalations can help you bring your cortisol levels back to normal again, decreasing physical feelings of anxiety.

Another great benefit of purposefully controlling your breath is that you learn to pay attention to your breathing. This awareness is crucial during stressful moments since being able to observe when your breathing pattern is changing to become faster and shallower helps you notice your anxiety levels increasing, empowering you to take action to self-regulate. You also learn to shift your attention to the present moment, making it easier to find calm and clarity in the moment.

Breathing exercises, like the two discussed below, are effective strategies for relieving stress since they can directly impact your body's stress response systems.

### *Diaphragmatic Breathing*

This technique is also called "abdominal, or belly, breathing." When your diaphragm is allowed to fully contract and relax, large amounts of air can enter and exit your lungs, encouraging more oxygen to be absorbed and carbon dioxide to be effectively expelled. The easiest way to determine if you're breathing with your diaphragm is to notice whether your abdomen expands during inhalation and contracts during exhalation.

The following instructions will help you practice diaphragmatic breathing:

1. Take a seat in a chair, on your bed, or on a blanket on the floor.
2. Take a regular breath while paying attention to how your body feels.
    a. Notice any areas of tension.
    b. Based on this, rate your feelings of stress on a scale of 1 to 10—10 being the most stressed you've ever been and 1 meaning you feel calm and comfortable managing your stress.
3. Purposefully relax your shoulders, neck, and head.
4. Place one hand on your upper chest and the other just below your ribcage. This will help you feel the movement of your diaphragm as you breathe.
5. Take a slow, deep breath in through your nose, allowing your stomach to move out against the hand below your ribcage. The hand on your chest shouldn't noticeably move.
6. Start to tighten your stomach muscles before exhaling slowly through pursed lips, allowing your stomach to move back into its resting position. Again, the hand on your chest should remain as still as possible.
7. Repeat the cycle 10 times.

### *Box Breathing*

This method is also called the "square breathing" or "four-square breathing" technique. It is a simple exercise that involves inhaling and exhaling in a specific pattern, making it an accessible but effective relaxation strategy.

The following instructions will help you practice this technique:

1. Start by sitting or lying down in a comfortable position, like in the previous breathing exercise.

2. Purposefully relax your shoulders so they can drop to their natural position. Then, place your hands on your lap or your knees.

3. Breathe in for a count of four. Inhale slowly and deeply through your nose while you count in your head. Try to inhale for just over four seconds.

4. Hold your breath in your lungs without straining for another count of four seconds.

5. Exhale slowly for a count of four seconds. Be sure to control your breath as it leaves your lungs, and aim to exhale for slightly longer than four seconds. Longer exhales help your body understand that you aren't in danger.

6. Repeat this cycle for several rounds.

    a. You can start with four rounds before slowly increasing.

    b. As you become comfortable with the four-second count, increase it to up to eight seconds.

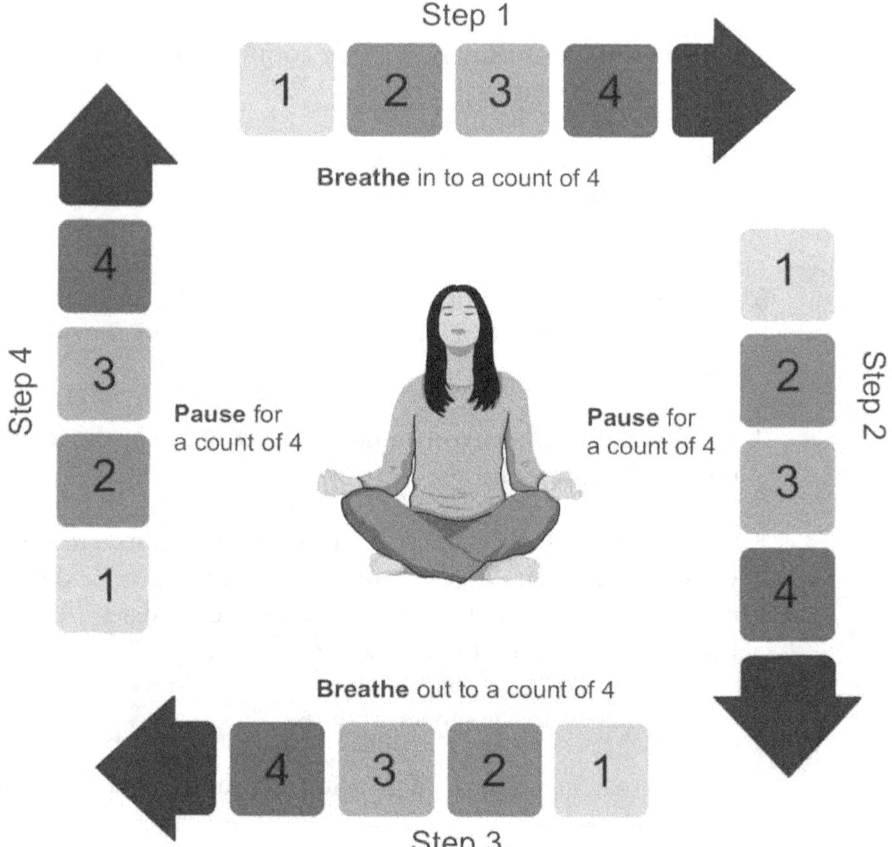
Step 1
1
2
3
4
**Breathe** in to a count of 4
Step 2
1
2
3
4
**Pause** for a count of 4
Step 3
1
2
3
4
**Breathe** out to a count of 4
Step 4
1
2
3
4
**Pause** for a count of 4

## *The Value of Grounding Techniques*

Anxiety often causes our attention to focus on the past or the future, making it challenging to stay in the present moment, which is where you need to be to complete the exam. Grounding is a coping method specifically designed to help you bring your focus to the present moment, allowing you to cope with and manage overwhelming and distressing thoughts.

This is a type of mindfulness strategy that allows you to redirect your attention from distressing thoughts and negative emotions to the immediate sensory experience. Grounding allows you to clear your mind, achieve a calmer emotional state, and choose positive coping mechanisms that are appropriate to the situation, allowing you to make decisions that won't cause further harm or distress.

Grounding is a technique I personally used to help combat my test anxiety. During medical school, I worked with a therapist who taught me to use a combination of my senses and my breath to ground myself. I was preparing for the United States Medical Licensing Examination (USMLE) Step 1—a type of standardized test that assesses the knowledge the student has gained during medical school and which takes place at a testing center. The centers for this test can be quite restrictive about what can be taken into an exam, which meant that I needed to get creative with my coping skills.

My first choice for an object that could help me stay grounded during an exam was a soothing stone or a smooth rock. Unfortunately, the testing center's restrictions prevented this. So, together with my therapist, we devised a solution.

I found a saint medallion that is often used in the practice of Catholicism. It was small and had an imprint of a saint on one side but was smooth on the opposite side, making it perfect for engaging my senses and keeping me grounded during the exam.

The metal was soft enough to pierce, so I turned it into a necklace that I could easily wear to the exam. When I felt anxious, triggered by indecision, or flooded with a lack of confidence about an answer choice, I would reach for my makeshift necklace, take a breath, and then rub the medallion; repeating this soothing cycle helped me get back on track for the test. Thankfully, there are many potential ways for you to practice grounding. You simply need to find what works best for you.

The following exercises are a few examples of grounding activities you could use.

### *Name Five Items*

This activity aims to help you calm your nerves and bring your attention back to the present moment. You can use the following steps to guide you:

1. Before your test begins, take a moment to look around you and identify five objects in the room or your vicinity.

2. Where possible, speak the name of the object out loud as you see it. Otherwise, mentally repeat its title three times before moving on to the next object.

### *Describe an Object*

By describing an object, you engage your mind in something constructive, helping quiet racing thoughts and keeping you grounded. This activity can be practiced as follows:

1. After settling into your seat, choose one object in your immediate surroundings.

2. Describe the object in detail in your mind. Focus on the object's color, texture, shape, and any other characteristics you notice.

### *Engage With Your Senses*

Engaging different senses, like touch and smell, is a great way to help you shift your attention and calm your mind. This was one reason why touching my saint medallion necklace was so helpful. Smelling specific scents may be especially helpful for reducing your anxiety. Lavender, rose, citrus blends, and jasmine are often great for calming the mind.

You could choose to keep a scented hand lotion in your backpack. This scent will be readily available, and being able to rub it on your hands before entering a test center means the scent is continuous as you work on your exam.

Pay attention while you rub your hands together, and allow the motion to soothe you. Be sure to take slow deep breaths so that you can enjoy the scent too.

You can repeat this exercise as needed depending on the type of exam you're taking and whether breaks are permitted.

### *Focus on an Object*

You may begin to feel anxious or become distracted during the exam itself. This is the perfect moment to use a physical object—like your pen, pencil, eraser, or any other small item—to ground yourself.

As you hold the object in your hands, pay attention to its weight, texture, and temperature. Notice these physical sensations so that you can help your mind refocus and shift back to your exam.

As you can see, there are many ways to ground yourself during a test. You can also take advantage of your mind's power to aid you in preparing for the test and combating stress.

## *The Role of Visualization Techniques*

We already know that the mind is a powerful tool. There are many strategies that rely on your mental power to help you prepare for your exams and cope with the stress that this situation triggers. Visualization is one of the most effective of these methods for combating test anxiety using your mind.

This activity is a powerful cognitive tool that uses your imagination to help you enter a calmer and more relaxed state. Essentially, you create mental images that help you alter your state of mind. The effectiveness of this tool has led to it being used for learning, sports performance, relaxation, and goal setting. I really love this technique because it allows us to use our minds to transport ourselves to a different space or time, making seemingly far-off goals, like succeeding on our exams, feel more achievable. But what does this practice look like in action?

### *Practicing Visualization*

Let's say you have a paper to write, but you're feeling overwhelmed by the amount of work it requires, causing you to struggle to come up with ideas. Visualizing the steps you could take will help you break the process into smaller actions and become more familiar with the steps you need to follow; this makes the paper seem less overwhelming to start.

For example, you might think to yourself that you will need to review the syllabus and confirm the due date and topics the paper needs to cover. You'll then picture yourself logging on to your course coordination program, opening the module details, reviewing the assignment details, and considering the materials you might use. Mentally rehearsing these tasks means that you will feel more prepared when the time comes to complete them.

Maybe, breaking your goal down into tasks like this will help you to realize that you should read a specific article or a selection of chapters from a specific book. After thinking about the materials you might use, you can imagine yourself sitting down to write the paper. Mentally walk through the steps you will need to follow. After imagining yourself opening up a new document, for example, you may visualize putting a few points on the page before the ideas start to flow.

While you may not immediately know everything your paper will cover, you do know that you are going to get it done and do it well. It can also be helpful to consider the areas where you may encounter obstacles or struggles. You may not know the solution yet, but picturing yourself overcoming any hurdles gives your mind the confidence and time to consider what you could do when you encounter them. Maybe, you could plan to speak with the lecturer or teaching assistant to get some clarity on something.

Then, imagine the intense relief you will feel once the paper is complete and you have submitted it. Take a physical sigh of relief if you need to; this will help you to embody the visualization and reinforce your own capacity to succeed.

Congratulations! You just completed a visualization exercise. As you can see, it isn't complicated. You're simply envisioning yourself successfully taking the steps to complete an activity. Visualization is a versatile technique that can be practiced for almost anything. Doing it multiple times a day, even during the task, can help you remove the uncertainty that often arises during situations that trigger anxiety.

Your conscious mind truly is powerful, but you can only benefit from it if you actively use it. Take note that consciously engaging in practices like visualization also helps your mind work on solutions to anticipated problems while you sleep, providing you with further benefits.

***Scenario Example***

To help you understand how you might practice visualization for a test, I'll walk you through the process I used to help a patient of mine who was preparing for a medical board exam.

She had taken the exam before but didn't pass, and this contributed to her anxiety. While she didn't think that she would feel anxious about going to the testing center, I wanted to ensure that we optimized all opportunities for helping her approach her exam calmly and confidently.

We started by visualizing the test day from the moment she would wake up. She planned to get up at 6 a.m. before getting dressed and taking her dog for a walk. She knew that she had a tendency to feel quite queasy on test days, so she planned a nourishing but uncomplicated breakfast.

Since she lived in a large city, she thought it would be helpful if she took an Uber to her exam. She knew she wouldn't want to talk to the driver on the day, so we imagined that she would offer them a polite greeting before communicating that she'd like to drive in silence. We also visualized the route from her neighborhood to the testing facility.

At this point, I decided that googling some images of the test site would help deepen the visualization practice. Since we were meeting virtually, I shared my screen with her. We looked at the entrance to the facility and could see the lobby and elevator. There were no other images available, so we used our minds to imagine the waiting room, as well as the desk and seat where she would take the test.

We anticipated how she might feel if she got stuck and what she would do if that happened. We also practiced a relaxation technique together to visualize how she would implement coping skills in the testing center if experiencing slight panic after encountering a difficult question. Finally, we imagined the exhaustion and confidence she would feel as she left the exam.

After she took the exam, she was grateful that we had practiced this visualization activity. It helped her feel more comfortable and confident about her abilities on the day. You can do this too!

Visualization is a great way to help you work through challenges, manage your emotions, and prepare yourself effectively. By knowing what will happen and when, you increase your confidence and help yourself find comfort during a situation that was previously filled with uncertainty.

## Step 5: Calming Your Nervous System

Since test anxiety affects your mind and body, the methods you use to calm yourself need to cater to both your mental and physical well-being. There are many strategies you could use, but breathing exercises, grounding techniques, and visualization are often the most effective methods.

These practices are valuable in situations other than exams too. For example, when you're in a lecture, giving a presentation, or working on an assignment, you can use these exercises to help you combat any anxiety or stress that may arise.

To master the ability to overcome test anxiety, simply practice these activities as they've been set out in this chapter. When you practice these exercises in different circumstances and sequences, you become more adept at applying them in any situation.

These exercises allow you to use the power of your mind, your senses, and your breath to calm your nervous system. As a result, they will be beneficial regardless of whether you practice them on their own or in a specific sequence. The key element is to become as familiar with their application as possible *before* you need to use them to pull yourself out of a crisis.

Be sure to check out our YouTube channel for additional videos that you can use to guide your breathing and develop your mindfulness when managing test anxiety: www.youtube.com/@collegepsychiatrist

## Key Takeaways

While you have the tools needed to help you calm your mind when you feel anxious, it's also important that you develop the skills needed for full-body relaxation. Coping skills are the best way to achieve this since they help you effectively and safely manage emotions, difficult situations, and stress.

Deep breathing exercises, visualization, and grounding are three techniques that have the ability to specifically calm your nervous system. And when this system is calm, you'll be able to give any test your full attention, helping you achieve academic success.

By developing healthy coping skills, you build your resilience. This is crucial for ensuring you're able to effectively navigate academic and life challenges, while also giving yourself room to grow.

Now, it's time for us to take a look at additional practices you can use to help you effectively manage your test anxiety.

## Chapter 6:

# Implementing Lifestyle Changes

The tools and strategies that we've covered throughout this book form part of cognitive behavior therapy (CBT). As an evidence-based, therapeutic framework, CBT emphasizes the connection between our thoughts, behaviors, and emotions. In other words: Your thoughts can impact your emotions, which affect how you react in a situation.

By helping you to take conscious control of this feedback loop, CBT truly is a beneficial activity that not only helps you manage stress and anxiety in a healthy and safe way but also maximizes your opportunities for success in all areas of your life.

As we move on to the final step in managing test anxiety, we need to look at additional lifestyle strategies that may benefit you further by ensuring you take care of your overall well-being. First, however, it's helpful to understand how the strategies we've already covered come together to form the CBT triangle.

## The CBT Triangle

At this point of your journey, you've already explored the most important connections in CBT. You learned how to identify your symptoms of test anxiety and how they may affect you. Then, you studied your negative core beliefs and thoughts so that you could begin implementing strategies that would help you change them into positive and life-giving thoughts. By taking good care of your mind, you could move on to learning how to calm your body.

The CBT triangle acts as a visual representation of the impact that your thoughts have on your emotions and behaviors. The tip of the triangle represents your thoughts, the bottom right of the triangle represents your feelings, and the bottom left of the triangle represents your behavior. If you work well with visual aids, you could draw a recreation of this triangle to quickly refer to when you feel anxious. This can make it easier for you to address your anxiety when you feel overwhelmed and your mind is clouded.

This image can remind you to

- identify the thoughts you have when you feel anxious.
- notice how you feel when these thoughts arise.
- be aware of how your behavior is affected by your thoughts and emotions.

Since we've already addressed the strategies and tools you could use to help you during this process, we're now going to move on to a few additional behaviors that could support you in reaching your goals. These activities allow you to focus on your overall well-being, forming part of what is called "integrative psychiatry."

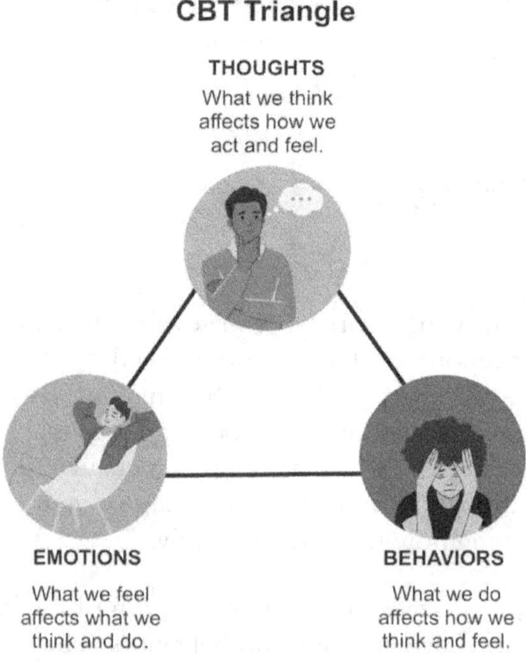

### *The Role of Integrative Psychiatry*

Integrative psychiatry considers your individual biology, history, and needs. As a holistic approach, this practice can help mental health professionals create comprehensive custom treatment plans that incorporate complementary and alternative therapies, in addition to traditional psychiatric treatments. This allows them to treat the whole person and not just the symptoms or condition.

This kind of psychiatry resonates deeply with me. My paternal grandmother is from the American South, and she and her six siblings relied on home remedies when Western medicine wasn't readily available to them. She would often tell me about the herbs they would use from their garden to treat a variety of ailments. I also grew up surrounded by books on complementary medicine in her library. So, incorporating elements of integrative psychiatry into my practice feels like a deep homage to my ancestors.

In this chapter, I'll also draw on my learning from the Integrative Psychiatry program at the University of Arizona that was led by two brilliant women, Dr. Noshene Ranjbar and Dr. Amelia Villagomez, to discuss the components of this practice and how you can use it to help you manage test anxiety.

In the following list, you'll find the key components of integrative psychiatry:

- **Traditional psychiatric treatments:** Approaches like medication, psychotherapy (CBT and psychodynamic therapy), and other established psychiatric practices can be vital for helping you stabilize your mental well-being and manage symptoms.

- **Complementary and alternative therapies:** Nontraditional treatments—like the ones discussed in the rest of the list—are used in addition to traditional psychiatric treatments to treat the whole person.

- **Nutritional interventions:** Your dietary habits can play a vital role in your health as nutritional deficiencies can impact your mental and physical well-being.

- **Supplements and herbs:** Sometimes, the body and mind need some extra assistance. Minerals, vitamins, and herbal remedies can provide this support.

- **Mind-body practices:** You now know that activities like mindfulness, tai chi, and yoga can have a positive impact on your stress and anxiety levels.

- **Physical activity:** Regularly moving your body can help you get rid of excess energy, manage your emotions, and decrease symptoms of anxiety and depression.

- **Traditional Chinese medicine (TCM):** This is an ancient practice that utilizes activities like acupuncture and herbal remedies to manage health problems and balance your body's energy.

- **Functional medicine:** A single condition can impact the entire body, so it's important to identify and address underlying psychological imbalances in addition to the health condition.

- **Lifestyle modifications:** Taking steps to ensure you get quality sleep, move your body regularly, and manage your stress can have a positive impact on your mental and physical well-being.

- **Psychosocial interventions:** You don't have to do this alone. Seeking social support, getting involved in your community, and asking for help can provide you with valuable support in addressing your test anxiety.

- **Spiritual considerations:** If you are a religious or spiritual person, it can be valuable to integrate your spiritual beliefs and practices into your daily life in a way that benefits your sense of purpose and meaning in life.

Our aim is to consider how you could incorporate such practices into your life to manage test anxiety. We'll take a look at three interventions: nutritional strategies, aromatherapy, and sleep.

## Integrative Strategies Valuable for Overall Well-Being

Since we've already covered many strategies you can use to help you manage and improve the impacts of your test anxiety, we can now move on to additional beneficial techniques. Let's get started with food's role.

### *Nutritional Interventions*

Receiving adequate nutrition ensures that your body and mind can function properly. If you struggle with food sensitivities and gastrointestinal issues or don't get enough of the right nutrients, your mental and physical well-being may begin to suffer. This could also contribute to mental health conditions like anxiety and depression.

However, nutritional strategies have to be practiced in combination with other anxiety management techniques. Think of food as the fuel that provides your brain and body with the resources to effectively learn, focus, and enjoy life.

Current research has demonstrated that your brain could benefit from a healthy gut environment—which is achieved through various nutritional strategies—resulting in improved mood, better cognitive performance, and decreased anxiety (Barbey & Davis, 2023).

Keep in mind that since diet is complex and hugely influential to your body, it's best to first consult your healthcare provider before making major changes to your food consumption due to the impact these changes can have on your health, especially if you have food sensitivities or allergies.

Below, you'll find examples of nutritional strategies that you could use to help you support test anxiety management:

- **Eat a balanced diet:** When you're in college or work a full-time job, it can be difficult to maintain a well-rounded diet. Do the best you can by aiming to include whole foods like unsaturated fats, lean proteins, vegetables, whole grains, and fruits in your diet.

- **Increase your omega-3 fatty acid intake:** These fatty acids have a variety of health benefits, but we're interested in their ability to support brain function and decrease inflammation, thereby decreasing anxiety symptoms and improving depression (Naidoo, 2019). Fatty fish like mackerel, salmon, and sardines, as well as walnuts, flaxseeds, and chia seeds, are great sources of omega-3.

- **Increase your magnesium intake:** This mineral plays a vital role in the body, specifically the nervous system. Increasing your magnesium intake via supplements and foods like leafy green vegetables, legumes, whole grains, seeds, and nuts can help you decrease anxiety symptoms and improve your sleep quality by aiding muscle relaxation and blood pressure regulation.

- **Take a vitamin B complex supplement:** Folate and vitamins $B_6$ and $B_{12}$ can play an important role in overall brain health. Their role in the production of neurotransmitters that regulate mood means they can offer some benefits for managing anxiety. Eating avocados, almonds, meat, fortified cereals, leafy greens, fish, poultry, and eggs can also increase your intake of these vitamins.

- **Use prebiotics and probiotics:** Probiotic-rich foods, like kefir and sauerkraut, may also be able to decrease symptoms of anxiety by improving your gut health (Naidoo, 2019). This is because about 90% of your body's serotonin—the neurotransmitter responsible for your mood, focus, and ability to learn and remember—is produced in your gastrointestinal tract (Cleveland Clinic, 2022b). Prebiotics like asparagus, onions, garlic, and bananas can also benefit your gut's environment, leading to better mental health.

- **Increase your antioxidant intake:** Since oxidative stress—which can negatively impact your brain—and inflammation occur due to low levels of antioxidants in the body, increasing your antioxidant intake can improve brain health and may help decrease feelings of anxiety (Naidoo, 2019). Strawberries, blueberries, walnuts, green tea, black beans, kidney beans, dark chocolate, apples, prunes, spinach, and broccoli are foods rich in antioxidants.

- **Eat tryptophan-rich foods:** Tryptophan is an essential amino acid that plays a vital role in the production of serotonin—a neurotransmitter that affects sleep, memory, emotions, and learning. Therefore, eating foods rich in tryptophan could lead to fewer feelings of anxiety and improved emotional well-being (Gotter, 2023). Eggs, milk, peanuts, tofu, chicken, cheese, and turkey are a few foods that contain this amino acid.

- **Eat complex carbohydrates:** Unlike simple sugars, complex carbs are absorbed more slowly, making it easier for your body to regulate and balance your glucose levels. This means you won't experience any drastic highs and lows, allowing you to achieve a calmer and less anxious state of mind more easily. Complex carbohydrates can be found in vegetables, whole grains, fruits, and legumes.

- **Stay hydrated:** Water is crucial for activities like digestion, blood circulation, nutrient absorption, and brain functioning. When you don't drink enough water, you may find it more challenging to manage your anxiety since your brain's functioning is affected (Stanborough, 2020).

- **Limit your alcohol intake:** The quality of your sleep can be negatively impacted by alcohol. It can disrupt your sleep-wake cycle, causing the REM stage of sleep to be harmed. Additionally, conditions like sleep apnea and snoring may also be worsened, further contributing to poor sleep quality that affects your mental well-being and anxiety. Alcohol can also trigger a type of rebound anxiety once its effects wear off. So, minimizing your intake can make your anxiety more manageable.

- **Limit your caffeine intake:** Caffeine can impact your brain's regular functioning and lead to increased feelings of anxiety. While you don't have to completely eliminate it from your diet, it's still helpful to reduce the amount of caffeine you consume in a day.

- **Reduce your sugar intake:** A high sugar intake can affect your body's blood glucose levels, which impacts your mental well-being. For example, you may experience a more positive mood after eating since your glucose levels increase. But as you quickly digest simple carbohydrates, if you ignore your swiftly renewed hunger, you may experience a negative mood due to dropping glucose levels. A high intake of artificial sugars can also contribute to intense fluctuations in blood sugar levels, leading to mood swings and anxiety. To manage this effectively, decrease your artificial sugar intake where possible. Instead, opt for naturally occurring sugars like those found in fruits and increase your intake of complex carbohydrates, as we discussed earlier.

It's important to note that the above information is not medical advice. Before you begin taking supplements, probiotics, prebiotics, or making any other changes to your diet, first contact your primary care doctor. Supplements, for example, can have negative interactions with medications you may already be taking, and these interactions could pose a danger to your continued well-being.

### *Aromatherapy*

This ancient practice involves using essential oils (plant extracts) for therapeutic purposes like managing anxiety and promoting feelings of calm. This practice is useful as smelling certain scents can promote feelings of calm in your amygdala—the brain's emotional center.

A study conducted by scientists at the Institute of Integrated Traditional Chinese and Western Medicine supports the idea that aromatherapy has the potential to help manage and reduce anxiety. It found that both long- and short-term aromatherapy interventions can have a positive impact on decreasing feelings of anxiety, regardless of whether you are healthy or have an underlying health condition (Gong et al., 2020).

We'll discuss how to safely engage in aromatherapy below. But first, let's take a look at the essential oils that can best be employed to tackle your test anxiety. The following scents are ideal choices, as they have been shown to have beneficial effects for managing anxiety (Gong et al., 2020):

- **Lavender** is a relaxing scent that can help relieve stress and anxiety while also promoting better sleep.
- **Ylang-ylang** may help decrease anxiety, improve mood, lower heart rate, and decrease blood pressure.
- **Bergamot** is useful for improving your mood and reducing stress and anxiety.
- **Clary sage** can reduce feelings of anxiety and calm the mind. It may also act as an anti-stressor by decreasing cortisol levels.
- **Rose** is perfect for decreasing stress and anxiety by lowering blood pressure, cortisol levels, heart rate, and breathing rate.
- **Frankincense** has grounding properties that can improve your mood and decrease anxiety levels.
- **Chamomile** can create a soothing effect, making it easier to calm your anxiety.

Essential oils can be used on their own, or you can combine them for a specific purpose. You can use the following blends to help you achieve a specific goal:

- **Calming blend**

- 3 drops of lavender
- 2 drops of bergamot
- 2 drops of chamomile

- **Stress-relief blend**
    - 3 drops of ylang-ylang
    - 2 drops of frankincense
    - 3 drops of clary sage
- **Energizing blend**
    - 3 drops of peppermint
    - 3 drops of rosemary
    - 3 drops of grapefruit

***How to Use Them***

Inhalation is the most common and effective method for practicing aromatherapy; however, topical application via an aromatherapy massage or a scented hand lotion can also provide benefits. The following section provides examples of how you could practice aromatherapy.

***Inhalation***

- **Personal inhaler:** A portable inhaler containing your chosen essential oil is perfect for on-the-go relief.
- **Diffuser:** Add a few drops of your chosen essential oil to your diffuser so that the scent can fill the space you're working in.

- **Steam inhalation:** In a bowl of hot water, add a few drops of your chosen essential oil. Then, drape a towel over your head after placing your head above the bowl and inhale the steam. Be sure to close your eyes as the steam may hurt them.

### *Topical Application*

- **Massage:** You will need to use a carrier oil, such as coconut or grape seed oil, to dilute the essential oil so that it's safer to use. You can then use this mixture to massage any part of the body that holds tension.

- **Rollerball:** Mix a carrier oil and your chosen essential oils in a rollerball bottle. You can apply this blend to the pulse points found on your neck, wrists, and temples.

- **Bath:** Add a few drops of your chosen essential oil to a warm bath. This can create a soothing and destressing experience after a long day.

### *Room Spray*

1. Add water to a small spray bottle.

2. Add a few drops of a high-proof grain alcohol—at least 60% alcohol.

3. Add a few drops of your chosen essential oil(s).

4. Close the bottle, and shake well before every spray.

### *Safety Tips*

Due to the lack of regulation on the quality of essential oil products, as well as everyone's individual reaction to them, it is vital to take precautions when using essential oils for any reason. The following tips can be used to guide you:

- Never ingest essential oils.
- Never apply an undiluted essential oil directly to the skin:
    - Always use carrier oils if you intend to use essential oils on the skin. Carrier oils include olive oil, almond oil, jojoba oil, and coconut oil.
- Before using an essential oil, conduct a patch test to determine if you might have an allergic reaction:
    1. Add a few drops of the chosen essential oil to a carrier oil, and mix well.
    2. Place a small amount of this mixture on your inner forearm, and cover it with a Band-Aid.
    3. If you've experienced no reaction or irritation after 48 hours, the diluted form of this oil may be safe to use.
    4. If you notice any itchiness or irritation, immediately remove the Band-Aid and clean the spot well. This oil may not be safe for you.
- Always aim to purchase high-quality and pure essential oils.
- Individuals who have underlying health conditions, are pregnant or nursing, or are currently taking medications should first seek the advice of their healthcare provider before using essential oils.

### *Sleep*

Sleep is one factor that's always emphasized in healthcare of any kind because this time of day is when your brain does its most important work. That's why you should aim to get between seven and nine hours of sleep every night.

A consistent sleep schedule provides your brain with an opportunity to improve its performance, as well as your mood and health. Interestingly, science has found that sleep and anxiety may have a bidirectional relationship (Alvaro et al., 2013). This means that when you don't get enough sleep or your sleep is disrupted, your anxiety will be negatively impacted. Likewise, if your anxiety increases, then you may continue to struggle to get good-quality sleep, thus creating a vicious cycle.

Let's take a quick look at what happens while you sleep so that you can get a better idea of why this activity is so important:

- **Memory consolidation:** When you sleep, your brain processes information and organizes memories. This is when short-term memories are converted into long-term ones, so this process is crucial for improving your recall and learning abilities, which can lead to better academic performance.

- **Synaptic pruning:** Your brain improves its functioning and efficiency by removing unused and unnecessary synaptic connections. This helps your brain simplify your neural pathways so that they function better, resulting in improved cognition. By creating more space and improving neural efficiency, your brain will find it easier to learn, grow, and adapt to new and unexpected situations.

- **Emotional processing:** A lack of sleep can make it more challenging for you to control your emotions. That's because sleep—particularly the rapid eye movement (REM) stage of sleep—allows your brain to process and regulate your emotions. This helps manage your anxiety, stress, and emotional responses.

- **Neural repair and growth:** During deep sleep, your body releases hormones with the ability to support cellular repair and regeneration. This is vital for the repair and growth of neurons, which can help your nervous system recover from daily stressors.

- **Energy restoration:** When you go to sleep, your body replenishes its energy reserves that were used during the day. This ensures your brain will have enough energy to function properly and efficiently the next day.

- **Balancing hormones:** The production and regulation of hormone levels in the body occurs when you sleep. This activity is important since the hormones that are affected by sleep can influence your stress levels, mood, and appetite. Cortisol and melatonin—responsible for regulating your sleep-wake cycle—are two examples of such hormones.

- **Dreaming:** You experience vivid dreams during the REM stage of sleep. The purpose of dreaming is still being studied, but it is useful for processing emotions, solving problems, and helping you cope with difficult experiences, and it may benefit creativity.

### *Sleep Hygiene*

Whenever my patients come to me with sleep difficulties, I find that it can be helpful to review their bedtime routines with them so that they can begin practicing good sleep hygiene. Sleep hygiene involves streamlining the practices and routines you engage in before bed that affect the quality of your sleep. Good sleep hygiene promotes consistent, restorative, and uninterrupted sleep.

You can use the following principles to help you improve your sleep hygiene:

- **Keep a regular sleep schedule:** The best way to regulate your body's internal clock is to go to bed and wake up at the same time every single day, including weekends. This can improve your quality of sleep.

- **Create a comfortable sleep environment:** Evaluate your bedroom. Is it cool, dark, and quiet when you sleep? If not, you could use tools like earplugs or a white noise machine to block out sounds. Blackout curtains are great for keeping the room dark, or an eye mask can provide a similar effect.

- **Have comfortable bedding:** Choosing bedding that feels comfortable to you can be invaluable. It helps you feel safe and calm, making it easier to achieve deep, restful sleep.

- **Limit your exposure to light:** At least one hour before you go to bed, you should start decreasing your exposure to sources of bright, cold light like your tablet, computer, or phone screen. These devices emit blue light which can interrupt your melatonin production.

- **Create a pre-sleep routine:** The best way to tell your brain it's time to start winding down for sleep is to create a bedtime routine. This routine will be unique to you but may include activities like relaxation exercises, reading, or having a warm bath.

- **Avoid stimulants:** Avoid using or ingesting stimulants, like caffeine and nicotine, in the late afternoon, as they make it more challenging for you to wind down and fall asleep.

- **Limit your alcohol intake:** Alcohol can negatively affect the quality of your sleep.

- **Take advantage of physical activity:** Regular physical activity during the day can help you get rid of excess or anxious energy, making it easier to get quality sleep. But avoid exercising before bed, as this can stimulate the nervous system and make it more difficult to relax.

- **Consider your diet:** Avoid spicy, rich, and large meals for at least a few hours before you go to bed since they may cause indigestion and GI discomfort that can affect sleep.

- **Limit the number of naps you take:** Long and frequent napping can disrupt your sleep patterns and quality of sleep. Try to avoid napping if you can, but aim for short, 20- to 30-minute naps early in the day if you do need to rest.

- **Use your bed for sleep and intimacy only:** To reinforce that your bed is a place for rest, avoid using it for activities like working, watching TV, or eating.

## Step 6: Making Use of Integrative Strategies

There are many additional strategies you could choose to incorporate into your life. But the practices you choose and how you implement them will be unique to your needs and lifestyle. Here, we will review a few holistic activities to help you get started.

### *Nutritional Interventions*

Your diet plays a vital role in your overall well-being and can be especially helpful for managing anxiety. You were provided with several dietary interventions earlier in this chapter. To get started, pick one or two strategies that you know you can confidently use and begin incorporating them into your diet. Then, give it a few days before reflecting on how you feel to determine if they made a difference.

### *Aromatherapy*

I utilize aromatherapy using scented hand lotions or a diffuser. For my patients, I specifically developed a self-care box called *The TCP Coping Kit.* This kit contains everything you need to safely and effectively utilize aromatherapy for managing test anxiety. You can find this kit at www.thecollegepsychiatrist.com/college-coping-kit

### *Sleep Diary*

Sleep diaries are useful tools for helping you better understand your sleep patterns and the factors that may be affecting them. This daily log can provide you with valuable information when you're trying to improve the quality and duration of your sleep for managing anxiety and improving your well-being.

For this activity, you will need your journal and a pen. Then, use the following key components and table to guide you in creating your own sleep diary.

The terminology you may need includes the following:

- **Bedtime:** the time when you go to bed and try to fall asleep.
- **Sleep onset:** the time it takes you to fall asleep after bedtime.
- **Night awakenings:** the amount of times you wake up during the night.
- **Wake time:** the time you wake up in the morning.
- **Out-of-bed time:** the time you physically arise and get out of bed in the morning.
- **Total sleep time:** the total number of hours that you sleep every night. Calculate this by subtracting your wake periods from the time in bed period.
- **Sleep quality:** a description of the quality of your sleep that night.
- **Naps:** how many naps you took during the day, as well as their duration.
- **Daily activities:** the activities you engaged in before bed that may have influenced your sleep quality.
- **Stress levels:** a brief description of your stress levels during the day and before bed.
- **Medications:** a list of any medications or supplements you're taking that may be affecting your sleep.

Below, you will find an example of how you might log entries in your sleep diary. Remember that this is just one way of tracking your sleep, and how you journal is entirely up to you.

# Sleep Diary

| DAY OF THE WEEK | | | | | | | |
|---|---|---|---|---|---|---|---|
| DATE | | | | | | | |
| **Bedtime:** the time when you go to bed and try to fall asleep. | | | | | | | |
| **Sleep onset:** the time it takes you to fall asleep after bedtime. | | | | | | | |
| **Night awakenings:** the amount of times you wake up during the night. | | | | | | | |
| **Wake time:** the time you wake up in the morning. | | | | | | | |
| **Out-of-bed-time:** the time you physically arise and get out of bed in the morning. | | | | | | | |
| **Total sleep time:** the total number of hours that you sleep every night. Calculate this by subtracting your wake periods from the time in bed period. | | | | | | | |
| **Sleep Quality**: a description of the quality of your sleep that night. | | | | | | | |
| **Naps:** how many naps you took during the day, as well as their duration. | | | | | | | |
| **Daily activities:** the activities you engaged in before bed that may have influenced your sleep quality. | | | | | | | |
| **Stress levels** : a brief description of your stress levels during the day and before bed. | | | | | | | |
| **Medications** : a list of any medications or any supplements you're taking that may be affecting your sleep. | | | | | | | |

## Key Takeaways

Paying attention to your overall well-being when you want to manage your health or a mental condition of any kind is crucial. It allows you to address your body and mind's needs, increasing the effectiveness of any strategies you may use.

Combining traditional psychiatric treatments with complementary and alternative therapies is especially useful. Keep in mind that while you may still use supplements or medications, the goal is to treat your whole self. So, pay attention to your social, physical, spiritual, mental, and emotional states. They can provide you with great insight into how to effectively care for your overall well-being.

We also know that there are a variety of CBT strategies you could use and combine to achieve this full-body treatment. Since we've covered a lot of information, you may be wondering how you can bring it all together. Turn the page to find out.

Chapter 7:

# Putting Your New Skills Into Practice

Now that you've reached the final chapter, you will have completed all three points of the CBT triangle, as well as incorporating several lifestyle changes that will further support the management of your anxiety. This ensures you're set up for academic success regardless of what you're studying or the severity of your test anxiety.

However, you might be wondering how you can keep your momentum and continue putting your skills into practice after finishing this book. This chapter will provide you with several tips and strategies to help you stay motivated to practice the six steps.

## Taking the First Step

We've covered a lot of information throughout this book, so what's the best way to put your new skills into action? The truth is that there's no single right way to incorporate the strategies and tools into your own life. Remember that we all lead different lives, and you may be at a different stage in your life and academic career compared to another reader. You may also have additional needs or lifestyle considerations that you have to think about.

For example, your classmate may be balancing her academic career and responsibilities as a mother, while you may be working in addition to completing your studies. And even though you are both completing the same course, the way you incorporate the tools and strategies in this book into your lives will be unique to your circumstances and individual needs.

This is actually a good thing since tailoring the methods you've been provided ensures they work for you, and everything you need to do so successfully has been provided to you in this book. All you need to do is start putting your newfound knowledge and skills into action.

## *Getting Started*

You may feel anxious and excited about beginning to implement practices to manage your test anxiety. That's normal. What matters is that you get started despite any hesitation you may feel. Remind yourself that you don't have to be perfect to benefit from the six steps. As long as you do your best and follow the instructions and tips I've provided you, you'll easily achieve success.

Since you may need to make minor adjustments to the strategies in each step, it can be helpful to track what does and doesn't work for you, along with any changes you've made to a strategy, in your notes app or journal. You can also make note of any ideas you may have about applying a strategy in a different situation to meet your needs better.

These notes can help you create a plan of action that you can use during moments when your anxiety is intense. Since your mind may feel clouded or you might be overwhelmed in these circumstances, having a written plan—made up of your tailored versions of the six steps—can make it easier to practice them and decrease your anxiety again.

Below, you'll find a few additional tips on managing your time and staying organized throughout your academic career. These basic tips can be used as a starting point for planning your approach to every new semester:

- As soon as you've received the assignment and exam dates, begin creating your study plan for the semester.

- As you become familiar with the coursework and how long it takes you to work through activities, review your study plan and make adjustments.
- Either start or end each day by planning the tasks you need to complete. This provides you with a set of mini-goals that you can achieve each day.
- Consider setting realistic and achievable study goals for each week. They should consider your class schedule and other commitments. This can help you work toward a long-term goal of being prepared for exams.
- Create visual reminders—like wall calendars and lists of important dates—to help you stay on schedule.
- Use phone reminders, even if you have to set multiple, to help you keep track of starting assignments and beginning exam preparation.
- Allow yourself to take breaks and rest.

These are just a few ways to get started. But how do you stay motivated when you have stressful and busy days?

## Keeping Momentum

We all have an innate drive to pursue and achieve our goals. But your motivation levels can be affected by a variety of factors, like how much you want to achieve a specific goal, what you could lose if you don't work toward it, and the personal expectations that you set for yourself. As such, motivation can help you solve problems, change habits, overcome challenges, and pursue the things that are important to you.

However, it can be challenging to stay motivated when you're extremely stressed, feeling anxious, struggling with another mental health condition, or neurodivergent. Challenges like burnout can also affect your motivation levels.

Right now, you may feel extremely motivated to put all the knowledge you've gained into action. The thing is, you might not feel this way all the time. Hours of exam preparation, long sessions with study groups, and days spent on assignments can make it very challenging to feel motivated and invested in your academics every single minute of every single day.

So, the first step to successfully maintaining your momentum is acknowledging and accepting that you won't feel motivated all the time. This is normal. But how do you achieve academic success if you're not feeling motivated? Well, being consistent in your studies, taking care of your overall well-being, and managing your test anxiety can be more important than feeling motivated all the time.

## *Embrace Consistency Over Motivation*

You may have a tendency to put things off until you feel motivated, but that might mean that you never start pursuing your goals. This can also affect your academics and cause problems like cramming and procrastination. If you want to achieve academic success, you can't put off tasks like exam preparation until the last minute.

Valuing consistency over waiting for motivation allows you to continue progressing with your studies and succeeding. It can help you meet both your long- and short-term goals and ensure you don't fall behind on your coursework. However, this also involves being consistent in taking care of your mental and physical well-being. After all, you may find it more challenging to take part in your studies when your mind and body lack the energy to try.

Being consistent doesn't require any special tools or strategies either. You are simply showing up for yourself each day, even if you don't always have the same level of energy. Setting up small, realistic goals in the form of easy-to-achieve tasks each day can help you become more consistent in your academics and taking care of yourself.

Other strategies that can help you become more consistent include the following:

- Frequently assess and review your long- and short-term goals so that you can adjust them. This ensures you aren't overwhelming yourself and allows you to remain adaptable, especially since life can be unpredictable.

- Break larger tasks down into smaller activities, and start them earlier so that you have enough time to finish them. This may include breaking an assignment up into smaller sections so you still have time to attend study groups, classes, and work.

- See setbacks and challenges as opportunities to learn and grow. They may even be telling you that something isn't working and that you need to make a change.

- Schedule time for yourself. This can be challenging, but having time every week to do something that's important to you, other than schoolwork, can be extremely beneficial to your mental health and help prevent burnout.

- Hold yourself accountable. As a college student, you're being trusted to manage your academic responsibilities on your own. This means meeting due dates, preparing for exams, and attending study groups, for example. If you struggle with accountability, consider working with a mentor or asking a friend if you can act as each other's accountability buddies.

No matter your age or what you're studying, managing your test anxiety will allow you to have a memorable experience that you can look back on with pride. College is a place to learn and grow as an individual and student, so the world is your oyster when you implement the six steps to managing test anxiety.

## What's Possible and Other Tips

You now have all the tools and techniques you need to effectively manage and overcome your test anxiety. But you might be wondering what you can achieve by implementing these strategies, especially if you're pursuing a qualification that's very different from the medical degree that I did.

The good news is that all the strategies in this book are not only highly adaptable but also relevant to managing test anxiety regardless of the education you're pursuing. That's why I emphasized the importance of personalizing the six steps to your academic needs and lifestyle at the beginning of this chapter.

In this section, we'll take a look at what you could achieve when implementing the six steps, as well as a few additional tips to guide you.

### *The ACT/SAT*

The Scholastic Assessment Test (SAT) and the American College Testing (ACT) exams are standardized tests that assess your abilities to succeed with college-level coursework. Taking a preparation course for either the ACT or SAT, in addition to implementing the six steps we covered, allows you to enter either test feeling calm and confident. This can make it easier for you to achieve a score that's within several points of your goal, allowing you to be a competitive applicant for your favorite schools. And once you've gained admission, you'll get to study with brilliant professors and make the most of your college experience.

In the list below, you'll find a few additional tips on preparing for the ACT and SATs:

- Do your own research! There is an abundance of online resources and books that not only help you prepare but also provide you with the opportunity to take practice tests based on past exams. Choose preparation materials that work well with your own learning style and study preferences.

- Take practice tests. They help you familiarize yourself with the layout of the exam, the type of questions being asked, and the way they want you to structure your answers.

- Set aside enough time for study and preparation. You can't wait until the last minute. Preparing long before the exam can also help you decrease your anxiety about the test.

- Consider attending preparation classes or hiring a tutor. These resources can provide you with support, guidance, and feedback that can boost your confidence in your test-taking abilities.

- Sometimes, exams use specific vocabulary you may be unfamiliar with. Take time to familiarize yourself with this language so that you ensure you understand exactly what is being asked of you during the exam. This can be done using online practice tests and during preparation courses.

- Depending on the exam you take, you may have access to written formulas. However, it's still a good idea to study and understand these formulas and how they are used. This can save you time during the tests since you'll only need to quickly glance at the formula sheet to double-check information.

### *Law School*

If you've been a pre-law student, you've likely spent several years researching and understanding what is required to gain admission to law school and be a good lawyer. Like a good student, you've prepared for the entrance exam and know the content well.

After completing this book, you have the added benefit of managing and decreasing your test anxiety, allowing you to walk into the test with confidence and no sweaty palms. You'll breeze through the reasoning, games, and comprehension sections. The experimental section will be no problem either.

When you receive your test scores, you know they will allow you to shine along with your letters of recommendation. You can get into one of your top choices and be challenged by the intense curriculum. Yet, through the implementation of healthy coping skills and strong study tactics, you'll still graduate successfully. Post-graduation, you can take the job that suits you best and ace your apprenticeship, allowing you to become the best lawyer you can be.

Let's take a look at some tips that will help you navigate law school successfully:

- Get started on your assigned reading as soon as possible. It can be easy to fall behind and even more challenging to catch up due to the course load. Making summarized notes that you can later refer to will be very helpful for exam preparation.

- Take the time to read through your notes before each class. This not only improves your memory and keeps the information fresh in your mind but also makes it easier to participate and take more detailed notes during lectures.

- Attend every lecture. Your professors may cover information that isn't in the notes you've been given. Being at every class means that you can take note of this information and have it ready for review before exam season begins.

- Use review sessions to help you gain insight into areas you may be struggling. You may also be provided with tips for assignments and exams.

- Use practice exams to help you prepare, and seek guidance from your professors after noticing areas where you're struggling.

- If you've already completed tests and exams, review them and discuss your scores with your professors so that you can work on weak areas for the next exam. This can help you improve your overall performance.

### *Medical School*

Having to take the required general chemistry, organic chemistry, biology, and biochemistry classes may have already challenged your desire to pursue medicine, but you might still know that this path is definitely for you. Since you're always an excellent student, you have probably already taken the time to review what will be covered on the Medical College Admission Test (MCAT), including completing the practice questions. So, you definitely know the content.

After reading this book and incorporating something from each chapter, you've been able to visualize taking the MCAT calmly and with bold assurance. When your scores come back, they're going to act as a great complement to the rest of your application. As a result, you'll get into several schools and will need to choose the right one for you.

When graduation day comes, your white coat ceremony will be surreal. And as you pass through residency and fellowship, your academic anxiety will be a thing of the past. You'll easily become a competent and caring doctor that patients love.

Let's take a look at some additional tips for medical school:

- Stay on top of your work. You can't cram in medical school, and falling behind can happen easily. Do your best to create notes early, revise them before every class, and take more notes during lectures.

- Prepare in advance. The earlier you begin preparing for tests and exams, the more you'll benefit. This can also save you time and allow you to focus on weak points, get feedback from lecturers, and attend study groups.

- Don't compare yourself to your peers because you're not leading the same lives. Adjusting your study habits and techniques to ones that work best for you will be more valuable than trying to copy and keep up with classmates.

- Since medicine has many fields, it's important to embrace curiosity. You never know what unexpected direction you may be drawn in.

- Seek out help from mentors and professors. They can provide you with objective insight that may benefit you during exams.

## *Business School*

Picture this: It's been five years since you graduated from undergrad. You've worked in several roles at your company, and now, you're ready to apply to business school. After some research, you've figured out which school requires the Graduate Record Examination (GRE) versus the Graduate Management Admission Test (GMAT).

While there's some debate about which preparation course is best, you make your decision and go all in. It can be tough to study and work at the same time, but you're doing it. You've got the content down, and with the help of this book, you've visualized your success.

Test day comes and goes, and the release of your scores has led to you being accepted into one of your desired schools. New students are divided into their respective cohorts, and on your first class trip, you meet incredible people and feel inspired to pursue that particular area of business. Time only goes faster from that moment.

Graduation day arrives, and your test anxiety is like a relic from your past. You've finished school and joined (or started) a successful business that makes you happy.

Let's look at some additional tips for business school:

- Your school will have a variety of resources; use them! They can make preparing for assignments and exams much easier and, potentially, offer insight that you may not have been given during your classes.

- Business is about connection. So, get to know your peers, connect with your professors, and engage inside and outside of the classroom.

- Be open to feedback. It can help you navigate your coursework and offer insight that may be useful for exams.

- Manage your time effectively so that you have enough time to complete assignments and prepare for exams. As with the other areas of study, it can be easy to fall behind, and catching up may feel impossible. So, do your best to stay on top of preparation and coursework.

- Take time to prepare for every class. This includes doing assigned readings and reviewing notes.

- Join in on class discussions since they can offer insight that written notes aren't always able to provide. This can also prepare you for real-life scenarios where you would apply this information.

- It can be helpful to stay up-to-date on news and economic trends since they influence and shape the business world. This may even offer you benefits during exams and assignments.

While I haven't covered all potential areas of study or the exam types you may take, you can adapt these strategies and tips to suit your needs. Don't hesitate to read through each section and note in your journal the points that resonate the most with you. You can use them to help you create your own approach to the coursework that matches your learning style.

It's also crucial that you celebrate every victory throughout your academic career, regardless of how small or insignificant they may seem. After all, you've put in a lot of time and hard work to get to this point, and that deserves recognition.

## Key Takeaways

In this chapter, we looked at the final tips and strategies for building a memorable and successful academic experience. However, you can only achieve success by putting what you've learned into action.

While you may not always feel motivated, practicing consistency—in addition to the six steps for managing your test anxiety—can ensure you stay on top of your coursework. This makes it a lot easier to seek guidance and prepare for exams, allowing you to approach every class, assignment, presentation, and test with confidence in your abilities to succeed.

Remember that no one will be able to carry out your profession the way you can. But you have to conquer your academic anxiety and keep going so that you can bring your unique take on the profession to the world. So, decide for yourself who you want to be.

# Conclusion

On graduation day in the spring of 2005, things were not looking good for me. My GPA was terrible, and most of my mentors believed I wouldn't ever gain admission to medical school. They actually recommended that I pursue public health or another health-related field. But I refused to give up. I got help, and I listened to all the voices that were encouraging me because I knew I could make a unique contribution to this world.

As I prepared for medical school, I didn't yet know about my anxiety and learning difference or the impact they were having. Instead, I figured out a system that worked for me throughout my post-baccalaureate program at the Harvard Extension School. My GPA and MCAT scores improved, and I felt confident about applying to medical school. So, when I got to the Anatomy module, I knew that I could do it. I could rise to the challenge because I'd done it before.

You probably have a similar story. Maybe, you were the star student in high school and have even excelled in portions of college. But right now, the tests you're taking aren't showing what you're truly capable of.

I knew that getting help would allow me to make it through, and it did. Just like you're reading this book for help, I reached out for therapy and neuropsychological testing. These tools helped me persevere and earn my medical degree. And the tools and skills that I learned during these difficult times continue to serve me as I approach new challenges even after finishing school.

I want you to keep this in mind: The richness of your applications and the potential you have to contribute to your profession cannot be captured solely by your test scores. But scoring high enough does allow the admissions officers to see all of the other ways in which you shine. How do I know? Because this was my story.

My scores may not have been the highest, but they were enough for schools to look at me and see my potential to be a thoughtful physician. Sometimes, a look is all you need to get to the next step.

I know that if I hadn't persevered despite the challenges I faced or if I wasn't supported by my community, I wouldn't have been able to make an impact on the lives of all the patients I've served, including you. So, keep going, and know that I'm cheering you on.

From the moment you opened this book, you started learning how to manage and overcome your test anxiety. We covered a lot of information together, and you learned about my own battles with academic anxiety. While I did overcome it, asking for help provided me with valuable guidance tailored to my specific needs.

Taking a look at what test anxiety is and how it works helped you understand how you might be affected. After all, no two people will be impacted by test anxiety in the same way.

From there, we dived into core beliefs and how you can identify them. This allowed you to gain insight into how they influence your test anxiety. Using this knowledge, you learned CBT strategies to successfully change your mind so that your thoughts were more positive and beneficial.

But your mind is only one part of you, and your entire self can be impacted by your anxiety. So, you learned how to relax your body using additional techniques that are also based in CBT. The effectiveness of the techniques and skills you learned throughout the book were boosted and supported by integrative psychiatry practices that make up the final step to managing your test anxiety.

In the last chapter, we took a look at what could be possible when you consistently practice and implement the six steps to managing your test anxiety. As a result, you've successfully completed all three points of the CBT triangle.

You're walking away from this book with the ability to identify how your thoughts are impacting your emotions and how this impact may lead to specific behaviors that either benefit or hinder you. All that's left for you to do is put your newfound skills and tools into action and take back control of your academic career and future.

I truly hope that you've found this book helpful. If so, please consider leaving a review and sharing this book with others. If you're still feeling stuck, need a bit of extra help, or would like some guidance on working through a specific section, you can reach out to us for one-on-one help that's been further tailored to your needs.

One-on-one sessions can be beneficial since they offer an opportunity for screening and potential diagnosis of other mental health conditions and learning differences that may be affecting you. Together, we can then explore their management and whether or not you could benefit from prescribed medication.

Additionally, we offer an eight-week, one-on-one course that dives deeper into each topic covered in this book. To find out more about the course and our services, visit our website at www.thecollegepsychiatrist.com.

# References

*ACT vs. SAT, what's the difference?* (2024, June 28). IDP. https://www.idp.com/blog/act-vs-sat/#1

Algorani, E. B., & Gupta, V. (2023, April 24). *Coping mechanisms.* National Library of Medicine. https://www.ncbi.nlm.nih.gov/books/NBK559031/

Alvaro, P., Roberts, R. M., & Harris, J. K. (2013). A systematic review assessing bidirectionality between sleep disturbances, anxiety, and depression. *Sleep*, *36*(7), 1059–1068. https://doi.org/10.5665/sleep.2810

American University of the Caribbean School of Medicine. (2022, March 31). *Tips to help you succeed in medical school.* https://www.aucmed.edu/about/blog/tips-to-help-you-in-med-school

Barbey, A. K., & Davis, T. A. (2023). Nutrition and the brain—exploring pathways for optimal brain health through nutrition: A call for papers. *Journal of Nutrition*, *153*(12), 3349–3351. https://doi.org/10.1016/j.tjnut.2023.10.026

Berg, S. (2023, September 28). *What doctors wish patients knew about managing anxiety disorders.* American Medical Association. https://www.ama-assn.org/delivering-care/public-health/what-doctors-wish-patients-knew-about-managing-anxiety-disorders

Borman, G. D., Grigg, J., & Hanselman, P. (2016). An effort to close achievement gaps at scale through self-affirmation. *Educational Evaluation and Policy Analysis*, *38*(1). https://journals.sagepub.com/doi/10.3102/0162373715581709

Brazier, Y. (2017, March 20). *Aromatherapy: What you need to know.* Medical News Today. https://www.medicalnewstoday.com/articles/10884

Brinkman, J. E., Reddy, V., & Sharma, S. (2023, April 3). *Physiology of sleep.* National Library of Medicine. https://www.ncbi.nlm.nih.gov/books/NBK482512/

Brown, G. S. (2018, June 6). *Now is the time for integrative psychiatry.* Psychology Today. https://www.psychologytoday.com/za/blog/green-psychiatry/201806/now-is-the-time-integrative-psychiatry

Cenikor Foundation. (2023, May 27). *How asking for help can ease anxiety and other mental health concerns.* Cenikor. https://www.cenikor.org/resources/how-asking-for-help-can-ease-anxiety-and-other-mental-health-concerns/

Chapman University. (2023). *20 tips for success in law school.* Fowler School of Law. https://www.chapman.edu/law/student-resources/achievement-program/20-tips-success.aspx

Cherry, K. (2023a, May 3). *Intrinsic motivation: How internal rewards drive behavior.* Verywell Mind. https://www.verywellmind.com/what-is-intrinsic-motivation-2795385

Cherry, K. (2023b, November 13). *What is negativity bias?* Verywell Mind. https://www.verywellmind.com/negative-bias-4589618

Cherry, K. (2024a, June 7). *Why are you so anxious during test taking?* Verywell Mind. https://www.verywellmind.com/what-is-test-anxiety-2795368

Cherry, K. (2024b, June 23). *What is a mindset and why it matters.* Verywell Mind. https://www.verywellmind.com/what-is-a-mindset-2795025

Cherry, K. (2024c, July 7). *What is procrastination?* Verywell Mind. https://www.verywellmind.com/the-psychology-of-procrastination-2795944#toc-how-to-overcome-procrastination

Cleveland Clinic. (2021a, September 15). *Complementary medicine.* https://my.clevelandclinic.org/health/articles/16883-complementary-therapy

Cleveland Clinic. (2021b, December 10). *Cortisol.* https://my.clevelandclinic.org/health/articles/22187-cortisol

Cleveland Clinic. (2022a, January 11). *Vagus Nerve.* https://my.clevelandclinic.org/health/body/22279-vagus-nerve

Cleveland Clinic. (2022b, March 18). *Serotonin.* https://my.clevelandclinic.org/health/articles/22572-serotonin

Cleveland Clinic. (2022c, June 6). *Parasympathetic nervous system (PNS).* https://my.clevelandclinic.org/health/body/23266-parasympathetic-nervous-system-psns

Cleveland Clinic. (2022d, June 6). *Sympathetic nervous system (SNS).* https://my.clevelandclinic.org/health/body/23262-sympathetic-nervous-system-sns-fight-or-flight

Cleveland Clinic. (2022e, October 14). *DSM-5.* https://my.clevelandclinic.org/health/articles/24291-diagnostic-and-statistical-manual-dsm-5

Cleveland Clinic. (2024, February 29). *Oxidative stress.* https://my.clevelandclinic.org/health/articles/oxidative-stress

Coelho, S. (2021, October 29). *Feeling anxious? 7 coping skills to try.* Psych Central. https://psychcentral.com/anxiety/coping-skills-for-anxiety#next-steps

*The cognitive triangle: What it is and how it works.* (2020, February 10). Hudson Therapy Group. https://hudsontherapygroup.com/blog/cognitive-triangle

Cohen, G. L., & Sherman, D. K. (2014). The psychology of change: Self-Affirmation and social psychological intervention. *Annual Review of Psychology, 65*(1), 333–371. https://doi.org/10.1146/annurev-psych-010213-115137

*The college psychiatrist* [YouTube Video]. (n.d.). YouTube. https://www.youtube.com/@collegepsychiatrist

Crum, A. J., Santoro, E., Handley-Miner, I., Smith, E. N., Evans, K., Moraveji, N., Achor, S., & Salovey, P. (2023). Evaluation of the "rethink stress" mindset intervention: A metacognitive approach to changing mindsets. *Journal of Experimental Psychology: General, 152*(9), 2603–2622. https://doi.org/10.1037/xge0001396

Drillinger, M., & Lamoreux, K. (2024, July 26). *The 4 worst foods for your anxiety.* Healthline. https://www.healthline.com/health/mental-health/surprising-foods-trigger-anxiety

*8 tips on the life of an MBA student.* (2023, May 2). IQ City Unitedworld School of Business. https://uwsbkolkata.com/blogs/8-tips-on-mba-student-life/

*Essential oil skin patch testing.* (2014). AromaWeb. https://www.aromaweb.com/articles/essential-oil-skin-patch-test.php

*Essential oil sprays.* (2017, October 1). The English Aromatherapist. https://englisharomatherapist.com/aromatherapy-sprays/#

Estevan, I., Sardi, R., Tejera, A. C., Silva, A., & Tassino, B. (2021). Should I study or should I go (to sleep)? The influence of test schedule on the sleep behavior of undergraduates and its association with performance. *PLoS ONE, 16*(3), e0247104. https://doi.org/10.1371/journal.pone.0247104

*Exercise as an intervention of holistic medicine.* (n.d.). Physiopedia. https://www.physio-pedia.com/Exercise_as_an_Intervention_of_Holistic_Medicine

Felman, A. (2023, December 21). *What to know about anxiety.* Medical News Today. https://www.medicalnewstoday.com/articles/323454

Field, B. (2023, November 3). *Self-Sabotaging: Why does it happen?* Verywell Mind. https://www.verywellmind.com/why-people-self-sabotage-and-how-to-stop-it-5207635

*4 steps to overcome negative thoughts.* (2022, June 13). Mindfulness.com. https://mindfulness.com/mindful-living/overcome-negative-thoughts

Ginsburg, S. (2019, June 19). *What is cortisol and how can it trigger test anxiety?* Ginsburg Advanced. https://www.ginsburgadvancedtutoring.com/post/what-is-cortisol-and-how-can-it-trigger-test-anxiety#

Gong, M., Dong, H., Tang, Y., Huang, W., & Lu, F. (2020). Effects of aromatherapy on anxiety: A meta-analysis of randomized controlled trials. *Journal of Affective Disorders, 274*, 1028–1040. https://doi.org/10.1016/j.jad.2020.05.118

Gotter, A. (2020, June 17). *Box breathing.* Healthline. https://www.healthline.com/health/box-breathing

Gotter, A. (2023, April 19). *What is tryptophan?* Healthline. https://www.healthline.com/health/tryptophan#foods-with-tryptophan

HealthDirect. (2023, January). *Panic attacks and panic disorder.* https://www.healthdirect.gov.au/panic-attacks-and-panic-disorder

HealthDirect. (2024, August 13). *Motivation: How to get started and staying motivated.* https://www.healthdirect.gov.au/motivation-how-to-get-started-and-staying-motivated

Hersh, E. (2024, March 27). *12 healthy sleep hygiene tips.* Healthline. https://www.healthline.com/health/sleep-hygiene

Hogan-Werner, J. (2020, February 19). *How to ask for help if you're struggling with anxiety.* Grotto Network. https://www.grottonetwork.com/stories/how-to-ask-for-help-with-anxiety

*How to ask for help when you're struggling.* (2021, November 10). Pivotal Counseling Center. https://pivotalcounselingcenter.com/how-to-ask-for-help-when-youre-struggling/

*How to study for the ACT and SAT exams.* (2023, November 14). College Covered. https://www.collegecovered.com/plan/7-ways-to-prepare-for-the-sat-and-act/

Howe, L. C., Goyer, J. P., & Crum, A. J. (2022). "Harnessing the placebo effect: Exploring the influence of physician characteristics on placebo response": Correction. *Health Psychology*, *41*(11), 873–873. https://doi.org/10.1037/hea0001235

Hoyt, L. T., Zeiders, K. H., Ehrlich, K. B., & Adam, E. K. (2016). Positive upshots of cortisol in everyday life. *Emotion*, *16*(4), 431–435. https://doi.org/10.1037/emo0000174

*The importance of coping skills and better mental health.* (2023, February 17). The Juniper Center. https://www.thejunipercenter.com/the-importance-of-coping-skills-and-better-mental-health/#

*Importance of healthy coping mechanisms.* (2023, March 7). Fort Behavioral Health. https://fortbehavioral.com/addiction-recovery-blog/importance-of-healthy-coping-mechanisms/

The Institute for Functional Medicine. (2022, October 3). *The functional medicine approach.* https://www.ifm.org/functional-medicine/what-is-functional-medicine/

Jewell, T., & Hoshaw, C. (2023, May 19). *What is diaphragmatic breathing?* Healthline. https://www.healthline.com/health/diaphragmatic-breathing

John Hopkins Medicine. (2019). *Aromatherapy: Do essential oils really work?* https://www.hopkinsmedicine.org/health/wellness-and-prevention/aromatherapy-do-essential-oils-really-work

Keller, A. O., Litzelman, K., Wisk, L. E., Maddox, T., Cheng, E. R., Creswell, P. D., & Witt, W. P. (2012). Does the perception that stress affects health matter? The association with health and mortality. *Health Psychology, 31*(5), 677–684. https://doi.org/10.1037/a0026743

*Know a college student who could use a pick-me-up?* (2014). The College Psychiatrist. https://www.thecollegepsychiatrist.com/college-coping-kit

LaFrenierre, S. (2024, March 26). *Integrative psychiatry: A holistic approach to mental health.* Resiliency. https://resiliencymbmedicine.com/blog/integrative-psychiatry/

Maharaj, L. (2023, January 31). *The neurodivergent student's survival guide.* Medium. https://medium.com/@labmaharaj/the-neurodivergent-students-survival-guide-6bbf947be9f4

Mayo Clinic. (2024, April 2). *Electrocardiogram (ECG or EKG).* https://www.mayoclinic.org/tests-procedures/ekg/about/pac-20384983#

Moore, C. (2019, March 4). *Positive daily affirmations: Is there science behind it?* PositivePsychology.com. https://positivepsychology.com/daily-affirmations/#positive-affirmations

Morin, A. (2023a, May 9). *How cognitive reframing works.* Verywell Mind. https://www.verywellmind.com/reframing-defined-2610419#toc-benefits-of-cognitive-reframing

Morin, A. (2023b, December 5). *What to do when you have no motivation.* Verywell Mind. https://www.verywellmind.com/what-to-do-when-you-have-no-motivation-4796954

Mount Sinai. (2015). *Mind-body medicine.* https://www.mountsinai.org/health-library/treatment/mind-body-medicine

Naidoo, U. (2019, August 28). *Nutritional strategies to ease anxiety.* Harvard Health Publishing. https://www.health.harvard.edu/blog/nutritional-strategies-to-ease-anxiety-201604139441

National Health Service. (n.d.). *Psychosocial interventions.* NHS Wales Data Dictionary. https://www.datadictionary.wales.nhs.uk/index.html#!WordDocuments/6psychosocialinterventions.htm

The National Institutes of Health. (2016, March). *Understanding anxiety disorders.* NIH News in Health. https://newsinhealth.nih.gov/2016/03/understanding-anxiety-disorders

The National Institutes of Health. (2019, April). T*raditional Chinese medicine: What you need to know.* National Center for Complementary and Integrative Health. https://www.nccih.nih.gov/health/traditional-chinese-medicine-what-you-need-to-know

The National Institutes of Health. (2021, April). *Good sleep for good health.* NIH News in Health. https://newsinhealth.nih.gov/2021/04/good-sleep-good-health

National Institute of Mental Health. (2024, April). *Anxiety disorders.* https://www.nimh.nih.gov/health/topics/anxiety-disorders

National Institute of Neurological Disorders and Stroke. (2024, June 18). *Brain basics: Understanding sleep.* https://www.ninds.nih.gov/health-information/public-education/brain-basics/brain-basics-understanding-sleep

Newman, T. (2020, January 9). *What is nutrition, and why does it matter?* Medical News Today. https://www.medicalnewstoday.com/articles/160774

Nunez, K., & Lamoreux , K. (2024, August 9). *What is the purpose of sleep?* Healthline. https://www.healthline.com/health/why-do-we-sleep

Pacheco, D., & Rehman, A. (2024, May 9). *How memory and sleep are connected.* By Sleep Doctor. https://www.sleepfoundation.org/how-sleep-works/memory-and-sleep

*Part 5: Identifying automatic thoughts in CBT.* (2018). Cognitive Behavioral Therapy Los Angeles. https://cogbtherapy.com/cbt-and-automatic-thoughts

Raypole, C. (2024, January 29). *30 grounding techniques to quiet distressing thoughts.* Healthline. https://www.healthline.com/health/grounding-techniques

Resnick, A. (2023a, July 28). *How to spot and challenge your negative core beliefs, according to a therapist.* Verywell Mind. https://www.verywellmind.com/how-to-challenge-your-negative-core-beliefs-7554706#toc-consequences-of-harmful-core-beliefs

Resnick, A. (2023b, November 1). *Understanding Socratic questioning: A comprehensive guide.* Verywell Mind. https://www.verywellmind.com/socratic-questioning-8350838

Robboy, A. (n.d.). *Automatic negative thoughts and core beliefs.* The Center for Growth. https://www.thecenterforgrowth.com/tips/automatic-negative-thoughts-and-core-beliefs

Sanderson, C. (2023, April 8). *Change your stress mindset, change your life.* Medium. https://medium.com/wise-well/change-your-stress-mindset-change-your-life-2dcbaa34fb98

Sawchuk, C. N. (2024, May 14). *Test anxiety: Can it be treated?* Mayo Clinic. https://www.mayoclinic.org/diseases-conditions/generalized-anxiety-disorder/expert-answers/test-anxiety/faq-20058195

Scott, E. (2022, December 6). *Journaling to cope with anxiety.* Verywell Mind. https://www.verywellmind.com/journaling-a-great-tool-for-coping-with-anxiety-3144672

Scott, E. (2024, January 12). *Avoidance coping and why it creates additional stress.* Verywell Mind. https://www.verywellmind.com/avoidance-coping-and-stress-4137836

Selva, J. (2017, January 31). *Exploring the body-mind connection (incl. 5 techniques).* PositivePsychology.com. https://positivepsychology.com/body-mind-integration-attention-training/

Sharp, Y. (2023, October 5). *10 benefits and uses of frankincense oil.* Nikura. https://nikura.com/blogs/essential-oils/benefits-and-uses-of-frankincense-oil?

Somani, P. (2019, December 9). *Mindsets: Q&A with Dr. Alia Crum, Stanford Psychology.* Parul Somani. https://www.parulsomani.com/post/mindsets-q-a-with-dr-alia-crum-stanford-psychology

Sorensen, D. (2022, April 20). *How to ask for help.* Psyche. https://psyche.co/guides/how-to-ask-for-help-without-discomfort-or-apology

Stanborough, R. J. (2019, August 8). *The benefits of rose oil and how to use it.* Healthline. https://www.healthline.com/health/rose-oil#1

Stanborough, R. J. (2020, December 15). *Dehydration and anxiety: How to keep calm and hydrate on.* Healthline. https://www.healthline.com/health/anxiety/dehydration-and-anxiety

Star, K. (2022, March 10). *Using visualization to reduce anxiety symptoms.* Verywell Mind. https://www.verywellmind.com/visualization-for-relaxation-2584112

Took, N. (2023, June 1). *Synaptic pruning—why does your brain shrink as you sleep?* The Sleep Matters Club. https://www.dreams.co.uk/sleep-matters-club/synaptic-pruning-sleep

The University of North Carolina at Chapel Hill. (2021, September 28). *Keeping a sleep journal.* Campus Health. https://campushealth.unc.edu/health-topic/keeping-a-sleep-journal/

University of Tennessee Chattanooga. (2023, May 1). *An MBA survival guide: 13 tips for your first year.* Gary W. Rollins College of Business. https://blog.utc.edu/business/2023/05/01/first-year-mba-student-tips/

Vallejo, M. (2022, July 12). *The CBT triangle: What it is and how it works.* Mental Health Center Kids. https://mentalhealthcenterkids.com/blogs/articles/cbt-triangle

Vandergriendt, C. (2024, May 24). *What's the difference between a panic attack and an anxiety attack?* Healthline. https://www.healthline.com/health/panic-attack-vs-anxiety-attack#anxiety-attack

Victoria State Government Department of Health. (n.d.). *Breathing to reduce stress.* Better Health Channel. https://www.betterhealth.vic.gov.au/health/healthyliving/breathing-to-reduce-stress

Villines, Z. (2022, June 20). *Cognitive restructuring and its techniques.* Medical News Today. https://www.medicalnewstoday.com/articles/cognitive-restructuring#what-it-is

Villines, Z. (2023, February 13). *Core beliefs: What they are and how to identify them.* Medical News Today. https://www.medicalnewstoday.com/articles/core-beliefs#examples

Vinall, M. (2021, September 1). *How sleep can affect your hormone levels, plus 12 ways to sleep deep.* Healthline. https://www.healthline.com/health/sleep/how-sleep-can-affect-your-hormone-levels

Watt, L. (2021, July 22). *What are beliefs, core beliefs, limiting beliefs, and belief systems?* Liz Watt. https://lizwatt.com/articles/what-are-beliefs/

Werner, G. G., Schabus, M., Blechert, J., & Wilhelm, F. H. (2020). Differential effects of REM sleep on emotional processing: Initial evidence for increased short-term emotional responses and reduced long-term intrusive memories. *Behavioral Sleep Medicine*, *19*(1), 1–16. https://doi.org/10.1080/15402002.2020.1713134

Whelan, C. (2023a, July 13). *5 benefits of clary sage oil.* Healthline. https://www.healthline.com/health/clary-sage

Whelan, C. (2023b, July 13). *About ylang ylang essential oil.* Healthline. https://www.healthline.com/health/ylang-ylang

Whelan, C., & Fletcher, J. (2023, January 30). *About bergamot oil.* Healthline. https://www.healthline.com/health/bergamot-oil

Wooll, M. (2022, July 19). *Don't let limiting beliefs hold you back. Learn to overcome yours.* BetterUp. https://www.betterup.com/blog/what-are-limiting-beliefs

www.ingramcontent.com/pod-product-compliance
Lightning Source LLC
LaVergne TN
LVHW010838120826
845149LV00017B/3297

* 9 7 9 8 9 9 1 5 4 6 0 4 1 *